Endometriosis

Edited by Courtney Marsh

Published in London, United Kingdom

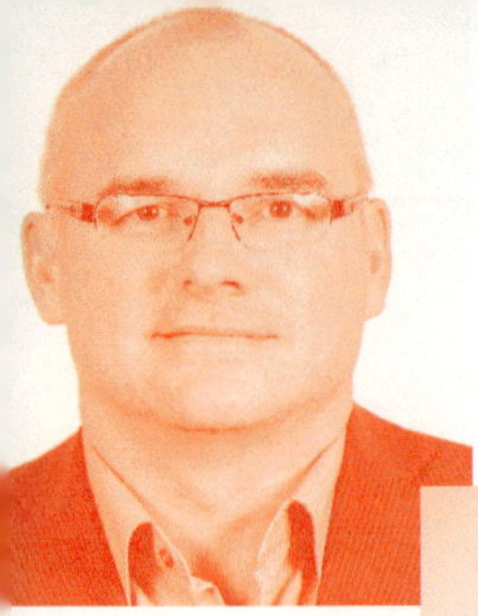
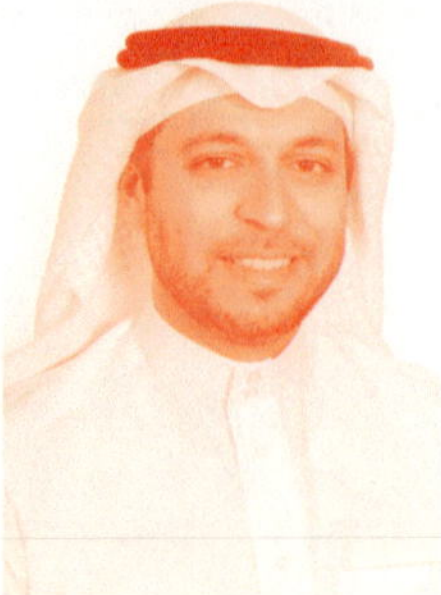
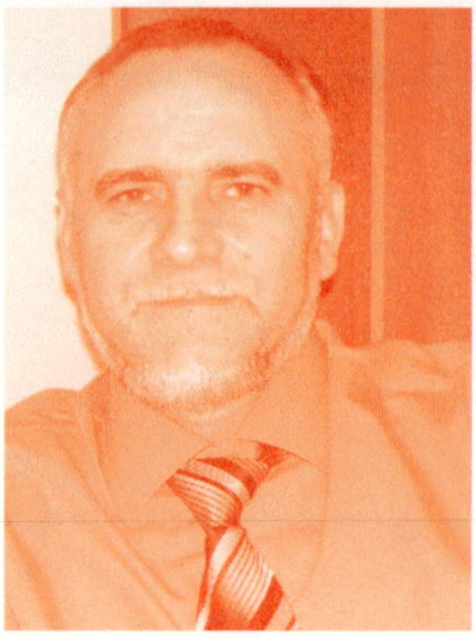
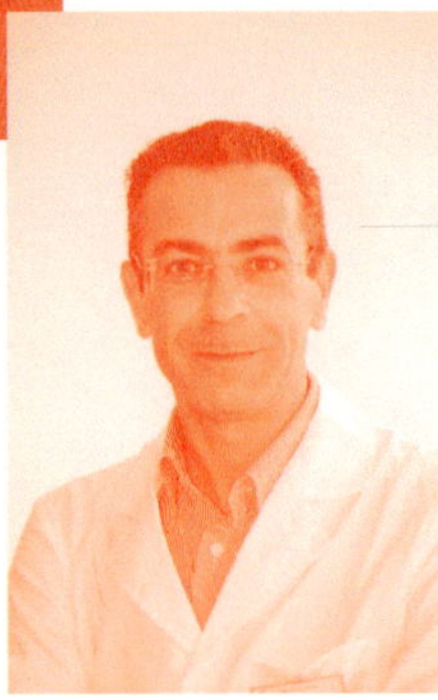
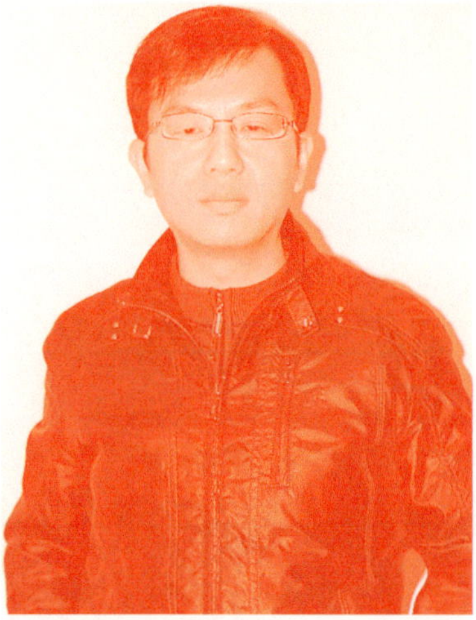
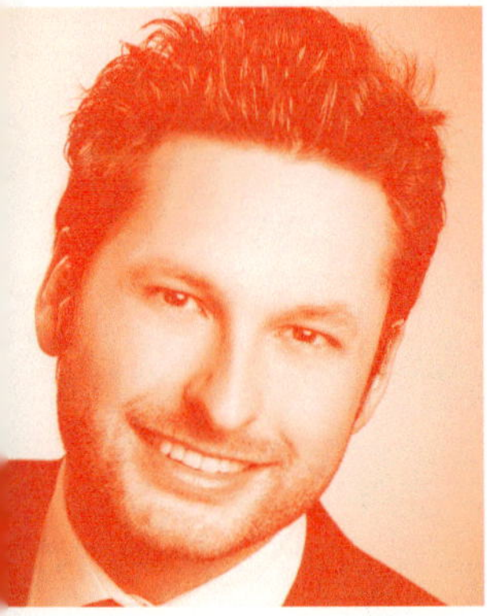
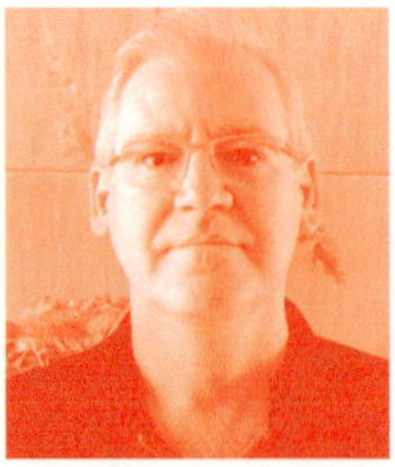

IntechOpen

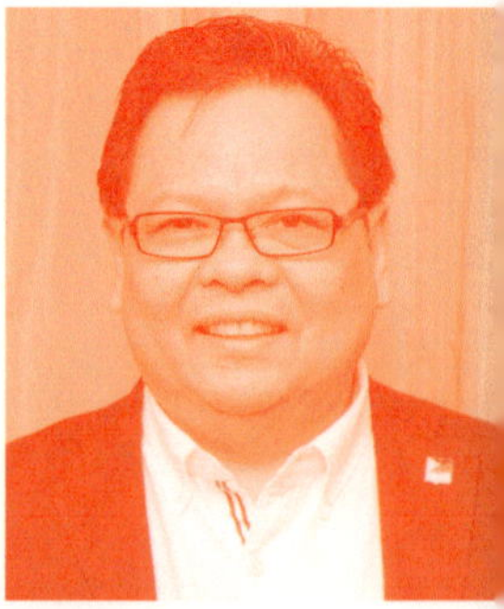
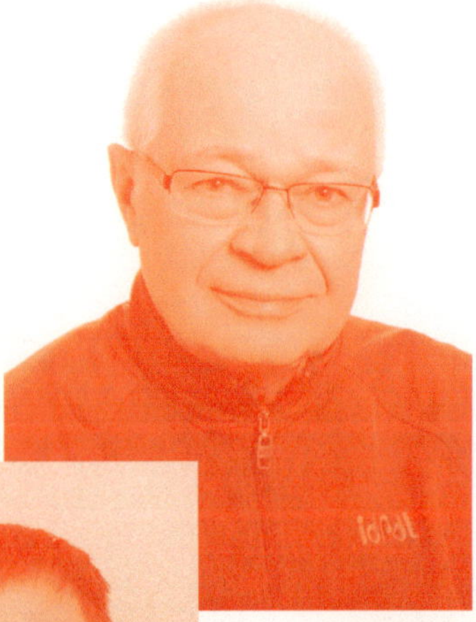
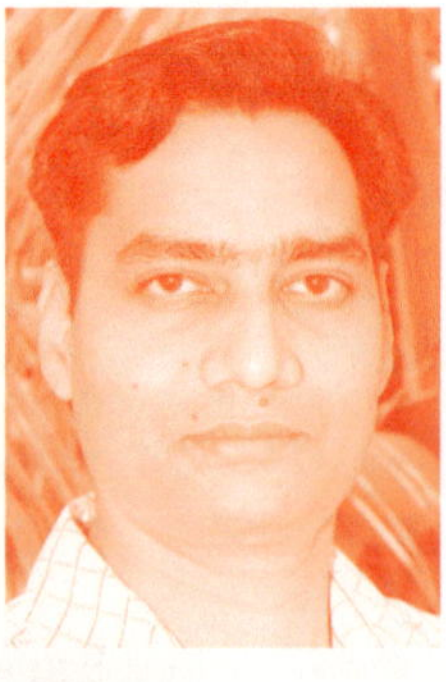
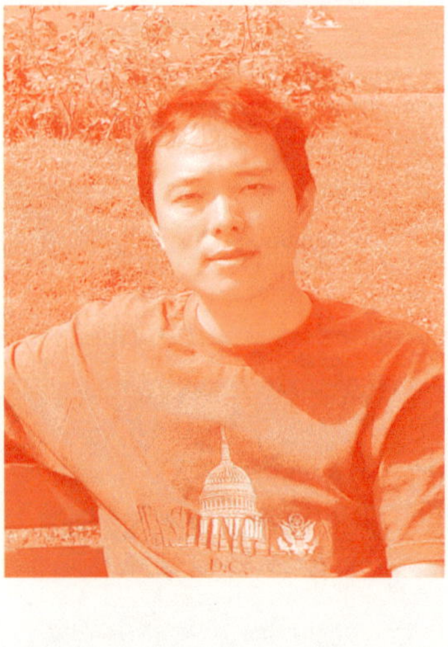
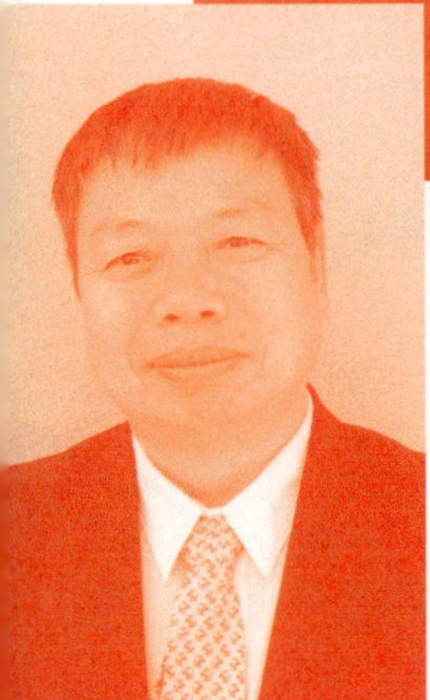
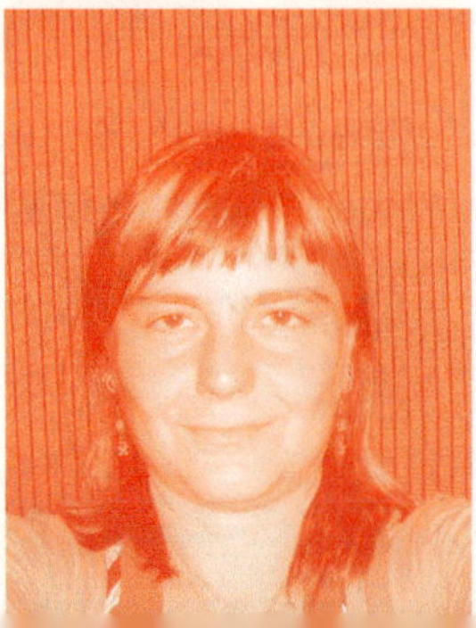

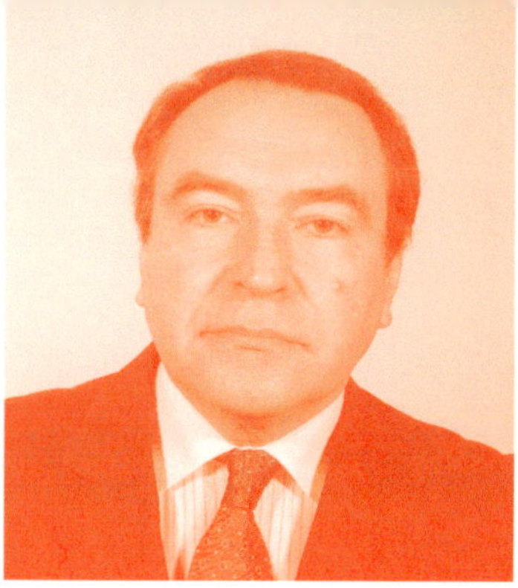
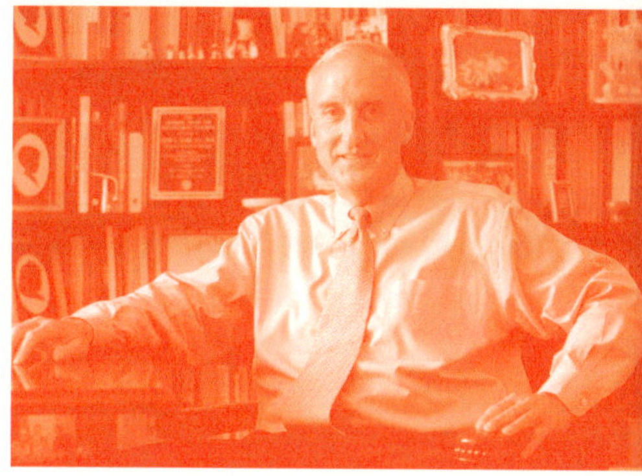
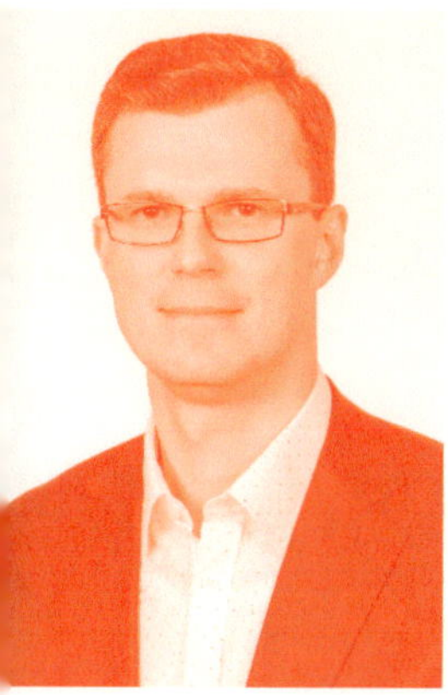
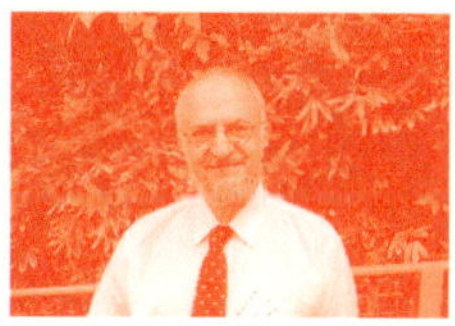
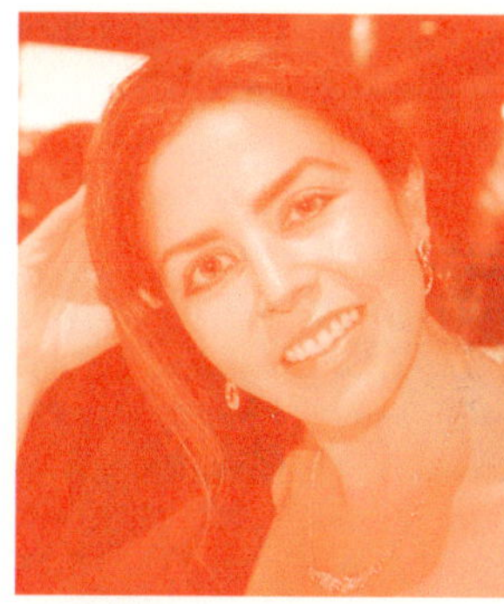

Supporting open minds since 2005

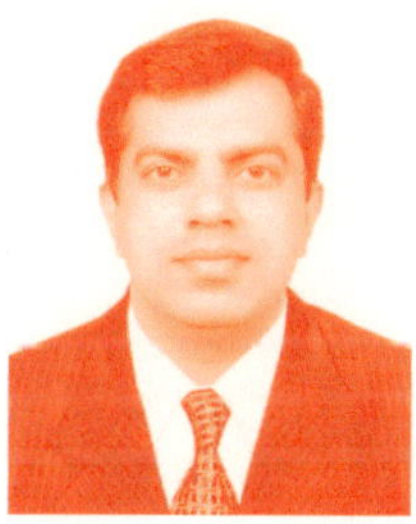
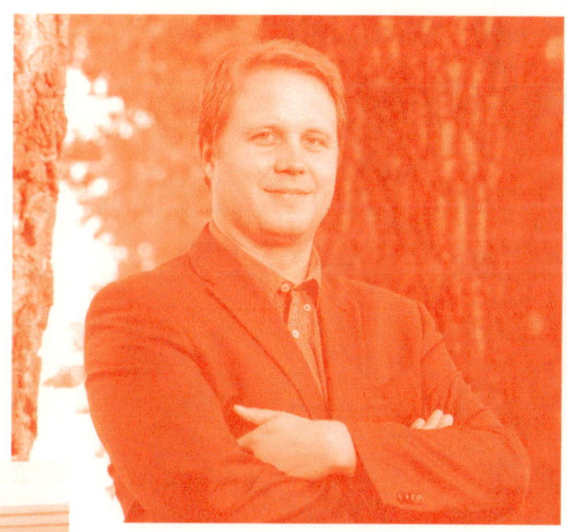
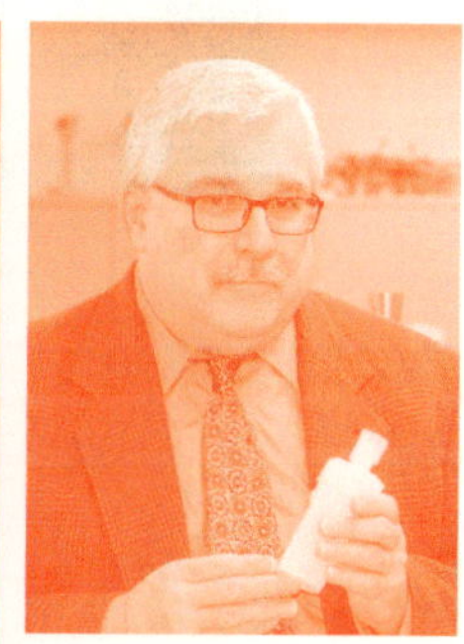
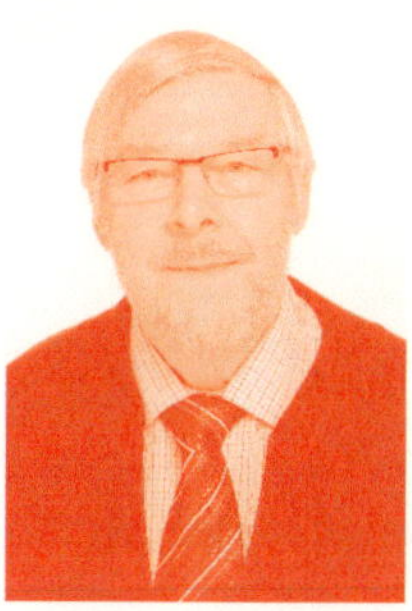
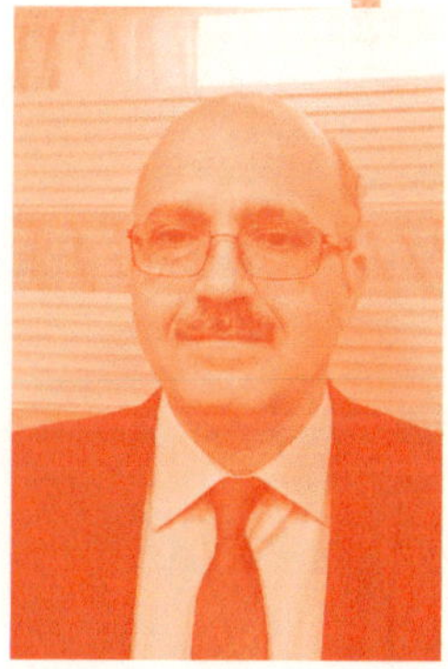
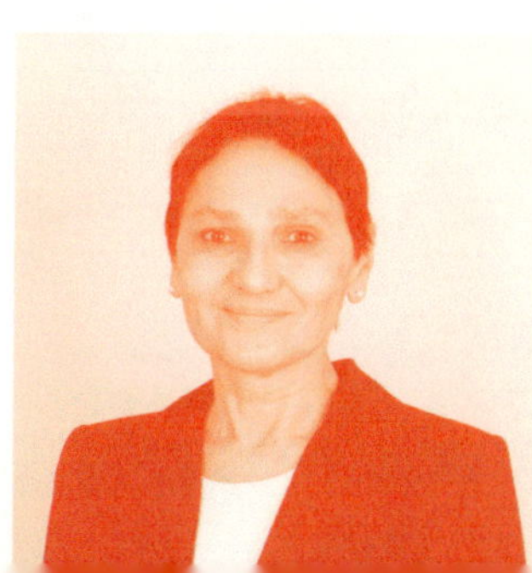
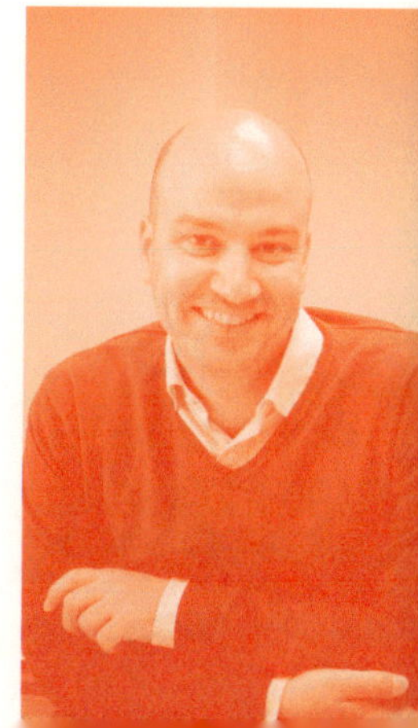

Endometriosis
http://dx.doi.org/10.5772/intechopen.87593
Edited by Courtney Marsh

Contributors
Wei Zheng, Warren Foster, Victoria Turpin, Anna Leonova, Sanjay Agarwal, Alexandr Popov, Alexey Koval, Irina Fedotova, Anton Fedorov, Svetlana Tyurina, Tamana Khabibullakh, Yang Xiaomin, Han Jun, Feng Pin, Yang Xiaojun, John Jarrell, Francisco Artacho-Cordon, Francisco M. Peinado, Luz M. Iribarne-Durán, Olga Ocón-Hernández, Nicolas Olea, Boya Deng

First published in London, United Kingdom, 2021 by IntechOpen
IntechOpen is the global imprint of INTECHOPEN LIMITED, registered in England and Wales, registration number: 11086078, 5 Princes Gate Court, London, SW7 2QJ, United Kingdom
Printed in Croatia

British Library Cataloguing-in-Publication Data
A catalogue record for this book is available from the British Library

Additional hard and PDF copies can be obtained from orders@intechopen.com

Endometriosis
Edited by Courtney Marsh
p. cm.
Print ISBN 978-1-83962-464-3
Online ISBN 978-1-83962-465-0
eBook (PDF) ISBN 978-1-83962-466-7

For EU product safety concerns:
IN TECH d.o.o., Prolaz Marije Krucifikse Kozulić 3, 51000 Rijeka, Croatia, info@intechopen.com or visit our website at intechopen.com.

Meet the editor

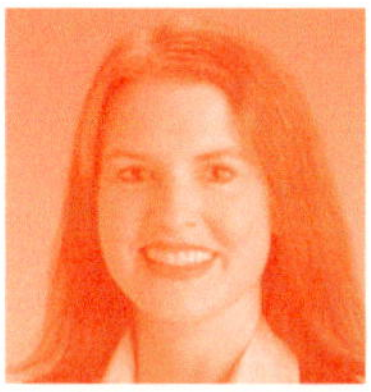

Dr. Courtney Marsh is Associate Professor of Obstetrics and Gynecology at the University of Kansas Health System and Chief of the Division of Reproductive Endocrinology and Infertility (REI). She attended the University of Kansas where she obtained both her undergraduate and medical school degrees. During medical school, she also completed a fellowship in Epidemiology at the Centers for Disease Control and Prevention at the National Center for Birth Defects and Developmental Disabilities. She completed her Obstetrics and Gynecology residency at Emory University and REI fellowship at the University of Michigan. Dr. Marsh's research focuses on improving fertility outcomes. Currently, she is funded by Garmin International, the Eunice Kennedy Shriver National Institute of Child Health and Human Development (NICHD), and the University of Kansas Medical Center.

Contents

Preface

Endometriosis is a prevalent disease affecting up to 10 percent of reproductive-age women globally. While we have made great strides towards our understanding of the pathophysiology of endometriosis, much is still unknown. We do know that endometriosis is estrogen-dependent and is mediated by immunologic factors. Defined as the presence of endometrial glands and stroma outside of the uterus, women may have debilitating symptoms including pain and infertility or the disease can be diagnosed incidentally at the time of pelvic surgery, making a determination of true prevalence particularly challenging.

In this book, we explore risk factors for endometriosis including environmental factors that are shedding light on this disease. We also investigate novel methods for diagnosing and treating pain related to endometriosis, which can be debilitating in some women. Conditions associated with endometriosis including adenomyosis, invasion of endometrial glands and stroma into the uterine muscle, and infertility are reviewed in depth. Finally, we look at treatment options for women with endometriosis ranging from hormonal to surgical. Together, we provide a comprehensive look at the diagnosis, treatment and risk of endometriosis to better inform practitioners in caring for patients with endometriosis.

Courtney Marsh
University of Kansas Medical Center,
United States of America

Section 1

Epidemiology of Endometriosis: Risk Factors and Environmental Contribution

Chapter 1

The Link between Environmental Toxicant Exposure and Endometriosis Re-Examined

Shay M. Freger and Warren G. Foster

Abstract

Endometriosis is widely acknowledged to be an estrogen dependent disease or unknown etiology. Recognition that environmental toxicants can bind with and activate the estrogen receptor, dysregulate steroid metabolism and, in some cases, act as anti-androgenic substances (phthalate esters) has led to proposal that exposure to environmental toxicants are associated with increased risk of endometriosis. Since our last review of the subject in 2008, the literature has expanded with several epidemiological and biomonitoring studies suggesting a potential association, whereas others have been unable to demonstrate a link between exposure and enhanced risk. Therefore, we carried out a systematic review and critical appraisal of the literature published over the past decade (2009–2019). The majority of studies found dealt with exposure to polychlorinated biphenyls (PCBs), dioxins, dioxin-like and non-dioxin-like compounds, bisphenol A and phthalate esters. Several studies suggest a potential association between exposure to environmental toxicants; however, important weaknesses in study design, methodology, and analysis together with many contradictory studies weaken confidence in these associations. Consequently, we conclude that despite a growing literature, evidence for an association between exposure to environmental toxicants and risk of endometriosis remains weak.

Keywords: endometriosis, endocrine disrupters, phthalates, bisphenol A, dioxin, estrogenic

1. Introduction

Endometriosis an estrogen dependent disease characterized by ectopic growth of endometrial glands and stroma outside of the uterine cavity. It is estimated that endometriosis may affect anywhere from 5 to 45% of all women [1]. Although retrograde menstruation has become the most widely accepted theory for the development of endometriosis [2], it cannot account for endometriosis in distant organs such as the lung and brain. Therefore, alternative explanations are sought.

While the cause of endometriosis remains unknown, it most likely arises from a multifaceted origin involving the interaction of environment and genetics [3]. Among the different hypotheses advanced, a growing body of literature suggests that environmental factors including environmental toxicants may play a role in the pathophysiology of endometriosis. Lifestyle and medication use point to a role for environmental factors in endometriosis. While alcohol consumption and cigarette smoking have been associated with lower endometriosis risk [4], developmental exposure to diethylstilbestrol and early life exposure to soy formula as well as alcohol consumption in adulthood was linked with an increased risk of endometriosis [4, 5]. Support for an environmental toxicant influence on the development of endometriosis surged with the report of endometriosis in rhesus monkeys treated with 2,3,7,8-tetrachlorodibenzo-*p*-dioxin (TCDD) [6]. Evidence of estrogen mimicry, dysregulation of steroid signaling, and immune modulation by environmental toxicants such as the persistent organic pollutants including the polychlorinated biphenyls (PCBs), dioxins and dioxin like compounds, pesticides, plasticizers (phthalates and bisphenol A), and some metals has led some to hypothesize that human exposure to environmental toxicants may play an important role in reproductive health including endometriosis [3]. Although a recent systematic review and meta-analysis suggests a possible link between exposure to chlorinated organic chemicals and endometriosis [7], we postulate that the role of exposure to environmental toxicants in the pathophysiology of endometriosis remain uncertain.

Potential associations between exposure to environmental toxicants and women with endometriosis have been equivocal with several finding positive associations [8–10] whereas others were unable to document an association [11–13]. Since our last review of the subject [14–17] numerous studies have emerged suggesting a potential link between environmental toxicant exposure and endometriosis [7, 18]. Herein, we describe a systematic review and critical appraisal of the recent literature linking exposure to environmental toxicants and endometriosis using a modified weight-of-evidence approach to evaluate the strength of potential associations.

2. Approach

We conducted a systematic review of the literature between 2008 and present, to capture publications since our last review of the subject [14, 17]. An electronic search was performed using PubMed and web of science between October and November 2019. The following search terms were employed: endometriosis and environmental contaminants, environmental chemicals, environmental toxicants, endocrine disrupters, dioxins, polychlorinated biphenyls (PCBs), phthalates, bisphenol A, and metals. Inclusion criteria included biomonitoring, epidemiology studies reporting chemical concentrations in women with endometriosis compared to a reference population and associated risk. We also included articles describing experimental animal studies and *in vitro* experiments designed to explore the effect of chemical exposure on endometriotic lesion survival, growth, and to elucidate potential mechanisms relevant to human health. Review papers, meeting summaries, commentaries were excluded as were articles written in languages other than English. Article titles were downloaded into an Excel spreadsheet and duplicate titles excluded. Articles meeting inclusion and exclusion criteria were decided by review of article titles and abstracts by both authors. Disagreements were resolved through discussion. Articles meeting inclusion criteria were printed in full and read by both authors.

3. Results

Our electronic search of the literature revealed 67 articles from which four articles with duplicate titles were excluded (**Figure 1**). We further excluded six

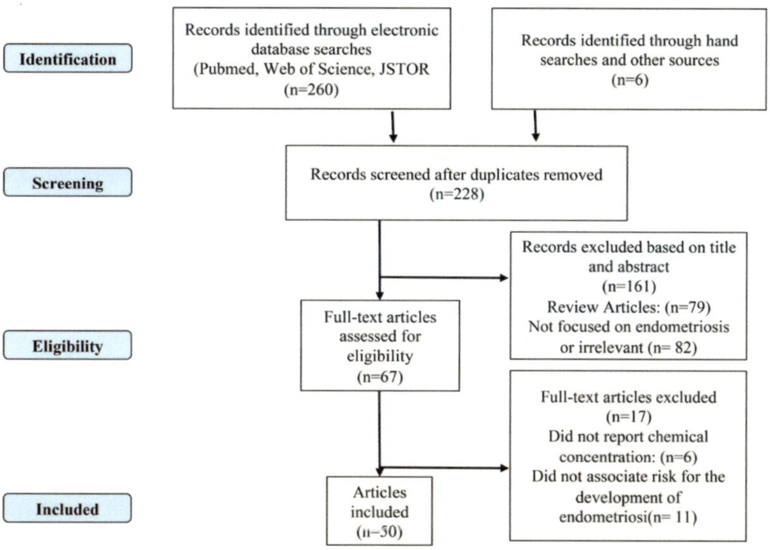

Figure 1.
Flow diagram summarizing the process of candidate article title identification in our electronic literature searches (PubMed and Web of Science) conducted between January 2018 and February 2019, screening, and article selection vs. exclusion. The number of articles included vs. excluded and reasons for exclusion are indicated.

review articles. An additional seven articles were excluded because they either did not report chemical concentrations or associated risk for the development of endometriosis. Consequently, 50 articles were retained for full assessment. The largest group of articles addressed the association between exposure to chlorinated organic compounds including polychlorinated biphenyls (PCBs), dioxins, and dioxin-like compounds with relatively few studies exploring the link between pesticide exposure and endometriosis. Of the chemicals with comparatively short half-lives relative to the chlorinated organic compounds and potential to disrupt endocrine signaling pathways, several reports linking phthalate esters and bisphenol A with endometriosis were found in our search whereas relatively few studies involving perfluoroalkyl compounds and metals studies were found.

3.1 Polychlorinated biphenyls (PCBs), dioxin and dioxin-like compounds

PCBs are one of the most widely produced chemicals worldwide, with millions of pounds being produced globally over the last decade alone [19] for use a coolants in electrical transformers. With 209 possible congeners, PCB toxicity is dependent on chemical structure. For example, non-ortho or mono-ortho PCBs are far more toxic due to the loss of chlorine atoms on the 2,2′,6,6′ of the benzene rings [20]. Due to their diverse structures, PCBs share similar characteristics to estrogen, allowing them to have both agonistic and anti-estrogenic activity [21, 22]. PCBs have been known to disrupt several organs and tissue types throughout the human body; with particular damage to the liver, kidney, and the endocrine system [19]. Our search revealed several studies primarily focused on PCB exposure and endometriosis and additional studies that explored the link between dioxin and dioxin-like compounds and endometriosis (**Table 1**). Since these compounds are frequently found together in human tissues, we will discuss them together.

In a pilot case–control study [24], involving 17 women (10 cases; 7 controls), superficial endometriosis was present in 90% of the cases. Of the 29 congeners measured in this study, both polychlorinated dibenzofurans (PCDFs) and

Authors	Cases vs. controls	Exposure investigated	Tissue	Outcome
Porpora et al. [23]	80:78	PCBs 28, 52, 101, 105, 118, 138, 153, 156, 167, 170, and 180	Serum	Increased risk of endometriosis for DL-PCB-118 (OR = 3.79; 95% CI, 1.61–8.91), NDL-PCB-138 (OR = 3.78; 95% CI, 1.60–8.94), NDL-PCB-153 (OR = 4.88; 95% CI, 2.01–11.0), NDL-PCB-170 (OR = 3.52; 95% CI, 1.41–8.79), and the sum of DL-PCBs and NDL-PCBs (OR = 5.63; 95% CI, 2.25–14.10) were all significant in case versus controls.
Cai et al. [24]	10:7	PCBs 77, 81, 126, 169, 105, 114, 118, 123, 156, 157, 167, and 189	Serum	PCB concentrations were higher in peritoneal fluid than serum. However, the total TEQ LOD and dioxin-like PCBs were not significantly different between women with endometriosis and the controls.
Trabert et al. [25]	251:538	PCBs 18, 28, 44, 49, 52, 66, 74, 87, 99, 101, 118, 128, 138, 146, 149, 151, 153, 156, 157, 167, 170, 172, 177, 178, 180, 183, 187, 189, 194, 195, 196, 201, 206, and 209	Serum	Several PCB congeners were associated with significantly lower risk (PCB 170 3rd quartile vs. lowest: OR = 0.5; 95% CI, 0.3–0.9) PCN196 (3rd quartile vs. lowest: OR = 0.4; 95% CI, 0.2–0.7), PCB201 (2nd quartile vs. lowest: OR = 0.5; 95% CI, 0.3–0.8; and 3rd quartile vs. lowest: OR = 0.4; 95% CI, 0.2–0.7) but not summed values (PCBs 170, 196, 201; OR = 1.3, CI 0.8–2.2) and estrogenic PCBs (OR = 1.1; 95% CI, 0.8–1.4).
Ploteau et al. [26]	68:45	PCBs 77, 81, 126, 169, 105, 114, 118, 123, 156, 157, 167, 189, 28, 47, 99, 100, 153, 154, 183, 209	Serum, omental, and peritoneal adipose	Significant correlations for PCB concentrations within the three biological compartments omental versus peritoneal adipose tissue were found ($p < 0.0001$). 137.1 vs. 147.9 ng/g l.w. for sum of 6 NDL-PCB. Adipose vs. serum: WHO-TEQ2005 DL-PCB = 3.6 pg/g l.w., sum of 6 NDL-PCB = 81.1 ng/g l.w.
Buck-Louis et al. [27]	190:283 and 14:113	PCBs: 18, 28, 44, 49, 52, 66, 74, 87, 99, 101, 114, 118, 128, 138, 146, 149, 151, 153, 156, 157, 167, 170, 172, 177, 178, 180, 183, 187, 189, 194, 195, 196, 201, 206, and 209.	Serum and omental fat	Higher concentrations in omental fat than serum. PCB-74, and PCB-156 in fat were inversely associated with the odds of an endometriosis.

Authors	Cases vs. controls	Exposure investigated	Tissue	Outcome
Martínez-Zamora et al. [28]	30:30	2,3,7,8-TCDD, 1,2,7,8-PeCDD, 1,2,3,4,7,8-HxCDD, 1,2,3,6,7,8-HxCDD, 1,2,3,7,8,9-HxCDD, 1,2,3,4,6,7,8-HpCDD, 2,3,7,8-TCDF, 1,2,3,7,8-PeCDF, 2,3,4,7,8-PeCDF, 1,2,3,4,7,8-HxCDF,1,2,3,6,7,8-HxCDF,2,3,4,6,7,8-HxCDF, 1,2,3,7,8,9-HxCDF, 1,2,3,4,6,7,8-HpCDF, 1,2,3,4,7,8,9-HpCDF, OCDF	Adipose tissue from the omentum	Dioxins and DL-PCBs were significantly higher in patients with deep infiltrating endometriosis; TCDD, PeCDD, PeCDF were the most significant $p < 0.01$ for each compound. PCB-126 (PCB-114 $p < 0.05$; PCB-156 $p < 0.05$; PCB-189 $p = 0.04$; PCB-126 $p < 0.01$).
Simsa et al. [29]	96:106	DLCs not specified	Plasma	DLC concentrations were marginally higher in patients with endometriosis (22.3±9.3 pg vs. 20.5±10.8 pg) and higher plasma levels of DLC were linked to a higher risk of endometriosis (aOR = 2.44; 95% CI 1.04–5.70; $p = 0.04$) adjusted for age. Moderate–severe endometriosis cases only (OR = 3.01; 95% CI 1.06–9.04; $p = 0.03$)
Vichi et al. [30]	181:162	PCBs 118, 153, 138, 170, 180, and total PCBs	Serum	With the presence of the GSTP1 wild type genotype, medium-high levels of PCB 153, high levels of PCB 180 and total PCBS were significantly associated with endometriosis risk (OR = 6.00; 95% CI, 1.88–19.18 and OR = 9.08; 95% CI, 2.14–44.4, respectively).

Table 1.
Summary of exposures and outcomes from biomonitoring studies designed to quantify the concentration of polychlorinated biphenyl congeners, dioxins, dioxin-like compounds (DLCs) and non-dioxin-like compounds (NDL) in women with endometriosis compared to healthy controls.

dioxin-like (DL) -PCBs showed no significant difference between the case and control [24]. However, both were elevated in peritoneal fluid relative to the serum, with the reverse seen in polychlorinated dibenzo-*p*-dioxins (PCDDs) [24]. Both PCDDs and PCDFs in peritoneal fluid were significantly associated with an increased risk of endometriosis [24]. Although a potential association was found, the small sample size, the authors did not adjust for other factors such as age that have previously been shown to affect endometriosis risk. Hence, confidence in the findings from this pilot study is low. In contrast, results of a case–control study [23] of 158 Italian women (80 cases; 78 controls), revealed that both non-dioxin-like (NDL)-PCBs and DL-PCBs levels were significantly elevated in women with laparoscopically and histologically confirmed endometriosis. An increased risk of endometriosis was found for DL-PCBs (PCB-118 [odds ratio (OR) = 3.79; 95% confidence interval (CI), 1.61–8.91], and NDL-PCBs including PCB-138 (OR = 3.78; 95% CI, 1.60–8.94), PCB-153 (OR = 4.88; 95% CI, 2.01–11.0), PCB-170 (OR = 3.52; 95% CI, 1.41–8.79), and the sum of DL-PCBs and NDL-PCBs (OR = 5.63; 95% CI, 2.25–14.10)). No significant associations were observed with respect to hexachlorobenzene (HCB) or to the sum of polychlorinated dibenzodioxins (PCDDs), polychlorinated dibenzofurans (PCDFs), and DL-PCBs expressed as total toxic equivalent quotients (TEQs). PCB-101, PCB-156, and PCB-170 were all shown to be statistically elevated, with PCB-52, PCB-118, PCB-138, PCB-153, and PCB-180 showing a highly significant difference. All four stages and endometriosis implant localizations (peritoneal, deep, or ovarian) were analyzed, with no significant differences detected. However, the lack of adjustment for potential confounding and failure to account for multiple comparisons are important limitations of this study. IN another study [29], DLC concentrations were quantified in plasma samples using the dioxin-responsive chemical-activated luciferase expression bioassay (CALUX). Blood samples were collected prior to laparoscopic surgery from women with endometriosis (n = 96) and control patients with a normal pelvis (n = 106). A marginal increase in DLC compound concentrations in endometriosis patients relative to controls (22.3 ± 9.3 pg, versus 20.5 ± 10.8 pg CALUX-TEQ/g lipid) was reported [29]. After adjusting plasma concentrations for age only, an increased risk for endometriosis was demonstrated for high concentrations of DLC (OR = 2.44; 95% CI 1.04–5.70, $p = 0.04$) and when considering moderate to severe endometriosis (OR = 3.01; 95% CI 1.06–9.04, $p = 0.03$). While the authors adjusted for age, adjustment for BMI, parity, and breast feeding was not undertaken. Thus, these results although suggestive must be interpreted with caution.

While several studies have provided evidence of a potential link significant associations between women with endometriosis and PCB levels could not be demonstrated by other investigators [25, 28, 31]. No significant association between PCBs and endometriosis risk was found in a study of 789 patients (251 cases; 538 controls); with 20 PCB congers measured in serum from surgically confirmed cases [25]. While the odds ratios (ORs) for several PCB congeners did show significant levels above and below the null; however, there was no specific pattern associated with endometriosis risk. Several PCBs were quantified in the serum of 473 women in an operative cohort (190 cases; 283 controls) and 127 patients from a general population cohort (14 cases; 113 controls), using omental fat in the operative cohort and serum in both [31]. Results were adjusted for confounding variables such as age, BMI, breast-feeding, cotinine, and lipids. Among the 35 PCB congers analyzed, geometric mean serum PCB levels were found to be inversely related in terms of risk in the operative cohort, with the opposite seen in the population cohort [31]. A similar relationship can be seen in omental fat, with sum PCB levels showing significantly higher levels in the non-endometriosis patients relative to the controls. Limitations of this study include the small number of women with endometriosis in the case population (only 11% of women had endometriosis), possible bias through the use of telephone directories, and use of controls without surgical confirmation of absence of disease suggest that results be interpreted with caution. The relationship between exposure to DLCs and deep infiltrating endometriosis (DIE) was explored in a case–control study of 30 cases and 30 controls [28]. Disease status was determined by clinical examination, magnetic resonance imaging (MRI), and transvaginal ultrasonography (TVUS), whereas the control population underwent laparoscopic surgery for adnexal benign gynecological disease. DLCs were analyzed omentum adipose tissue in both groups. The results suggest a significant increase of both dioxins and PCBs relative to the control, with the most toxic forms showing a significant difference (2,3,7,8-TCDD and 1,2,3,7,8-pentachlorodibenzo-*p*-dioxin [1,2,3,7,8-PeCDD]; $p < 0.01$) [28]. Furthermore, 2,3,4,7,8-PeCDF was also significantly higher and four of the most toxic PCB congeners (PCB 144, 156, 189, 126) had toxic equivalence values (TEQ) that were statistically higher in DIE patients [28]. However, no differences were seen when the data were adjusted for age, breast feeding, and BMI. Limitations of this study include small sample size, and homogeneity of the sample population [28].

A biomonitoring study conducted in France [26], measured the concentrations of PCBs in serum, peritoneal and omental adipose tissue of 113 adult French women with deep infiltrating endometriosis (DIE) (45 controls, 68 cases). There was a significant difference between omental versus peritoneal adipose tissue PCB concentrations ($p < 0.0001$). Similar trends were seen is peritoneal adipose tissue versus serum levels, with PCBs showing the highest level of significance in terms of concentration differences.

Potential gene–environment interaction among women with endometriosis was explored [30]. Specifically, the relationship between glutathione transferase (GST) gene polymorphisms PCB concentrations in a study of 343 Italian women (181 cases; 162 controls). Ability glutathione enzymes to regulate oxidative free radicals and thus oxidative stress and therefore genetic polymorphisms may influence tissue capacity to manage the damaging effects oxidative stress, in turn influencing disease susceptibility. No significant difference in genotype distribution (GSTM1, GSTA1, and GSTP1) between case and control patients could be elicited [30]. However, the GSTP1 wild-type with medium-high blood levels of PCB153, high levels of PCB180, or total PCB levels, showed a significant increase in potential risk, while GSTT1 null was negatively associated with the disease [30]. The potential association between five microsatellites and 28 single nucleotide polymorphisms among 10 dioxin detoxification genes (aryl hydrocarbon receptor (AhR), AHRR, ARNT, CYP1A1, CYP2E1, EPHX1, GSTM1, GSTP1, GSTT1, NAT2) was examined in 242 women (100 case; 143 control) from Japan [32]. Accounting for disease stages I-IV, BMI, and smoking, no significant association was seen between the polymorphisms and the contribution to the etiology of endometriosis. Taken together, these data suggest that genetic polymorphisms in detoxification enzymes do not modulate endometriosis risk.

Establishing a link between exposure to environmental toxicants and endometriosis using epidemiology and biomonitoring is difficult owing to challenges in diagnosis of endometriosis [33], lengthy diagnostic delays [34], and high prevalence of endometriosis in asymptomatic women [1] and thus the potential for misclassification error is high. Therefore, animal studies have been employed to better understand the potential hazard posed between toxicant exposure and endometriosis. Developmental exposure of mice to TCDD induced a progesterone-resistant phenotype in adult animals that persisted across generations [35]. Results of this study suggest that TCDD induced activation of the aryl hydrocarbon signaling pathway induces dysregulation of expression of tissue remodeling enzymes, and contributes to the inflammatory responses, cell migration, and proliferation seen in endometriosis patients. These data are supported by prior animal studies demonstrating PCB and dioxin effects in animal models of endometriosis [36–38].

Tissue culture studies have been employed to elucidate potentially important toxicant regulated mechanisms. PCBs have been linked to an increased estradiol synthesis and creating an inflammatory milieu through the production of interleukin (IL)-6 and IL-8 [39]. Primary cultures of endometrial stromal cells (ESCs) were treated with both DL-PCBs and NDL-PCBs. Dioxin-like CB126 treatment increased 17β-estradiol (E_2) biosynthesis in a dose dependent manner. CB126 exposure also increased 17β-hydroxysteroid dehydrogenase 7 (HSD17B7) as well as decreased methylation of the HSD17B7 promoter leading to an increase in expression. Inflammatory markers were also elevated in cultured endometrial stromal cells. Increased inflammation and E_2 synthesis were demonstrated in a mouse model of endometriosis [39]. Although PCB has shown to increase E_2 biosynthesis, combining 17β-Estradiol with TCDD showed a synergistic effect and induces M2 activation with macrophages co-cultured with ESCs. STAT3 and P38 phosphorylation in macrophages were also increased differentiation of M2 macrophages, leading to an inflammatory milieu [40]. Several studies also analyzed the impact of TCDD exposure on progesterone-dependent mechanisms. TCDD was found to induce cannabinoid receptor type 1 CB1-R mRNA expression in endometrial stromal cells and steroid-induced expression of the gene was inhibited. Through the use of tissue obtained from women with and without endometriosis, TCDD treatment-induced dysregulation of cannabinoid signaling, immune cell migration into the endometrium during embryo uterine attachment [41] and thus we propose could be an important mechanism in the pathophysiology of endometriosis. PCB was also seen to activate endogenous aryl hydrocarbon receptor (AhR) signaling pathway in immortalized human telomerase reverse transcriptase (hTERT) endometrial epithelial cell (hTERT-EEC), specific to time, concentration, and congener. The changes induced were modulated by changes in estrogen levels, in turn increasing cell migration by hTERT-EEC. Proteomic analysis also identified cell stress responses and metabolism markers (such as heat shock proteins (HSP) 27 and HSP 70) [42]. These proteins are both critical markers for the regulation of apoptosis and cellular stress response pathways. In another study [43] primary cultures of ESCs from both case and control patients showed that PCB-104 exposure affects cell migration, invasion and resultant gene expression. Treatments induced a significant increase in cell migration and invasion of ESCs. Enzyme-linked immunosorbent assays showed a time and dose dependent increase in matrix metalloproteinase 3 (MMP-3) and MMP-10 protein in ESCs, whereas MMP-2, MMP-9, TIMP-2, E-cadherin, Snail and Slug did not. MMP-3 contributes to the breakdown of the extracellular matrix and promotes tissue remodeling and migration [43]. The results from this study suggest that PCB-104 increased migration and invasion of ESCs through increasing MMP-3 and MMP-10 [43]. Taken together, results from tissue culture studies elucidate PCB and dioxin induced dysregulation of mechanisms potentially important in the pathophysiology of endometriosis.

In summary, several studies demonstrated a potential association between exposure to PCBs, dioxins, and dioxin-like compounds and increased risk of endometriosis; however, important study limitations decrease confidence in these study findings. Moreover, several studies were unable to evoke evidence of an association between exposure to these toxicants. While, animal studies are few, results from these studies provide evidence of biological plausibility. Results of tissue culture studies also provide evidence that PCBs and dioxins adversely affect mechanistic pathways important in the pathophysiology of endometriosis although the effective concentrations exceed human exposure. Consequently, we suggest that there is weak evidence linking exposure to PCBs and dioxin and DL-PCBs in the pathophysiology of endometriosis.

3.2 Pesticides

Chlorinated organic pesticides (COPs) resist degradation in the environment, are lipophilic and thus bioaccumulate in adipose tissues, and concentrations are biomagnified with increasing trophic level. Moreover, COPs are able to travel long distances and remain stable for several decades in the environment, and thus widespread human exposure to these chemicals has frequently been documented. Despite widespread human exposure, the relationship between pesticides and endometriosis risk in general are equivocal.

The concentrations of six COP levels were measured with gas chromatography and electron-capture, in blood samples of laparoscopically confirmed cases of endometriosis [44]. Results showed that aromatic fungicides had a five-fold increase in risk (aOR = 5.3; 95% CI, 1.2–23.6) when comparing the highest and lowest tertile after adjusting for smoking and serum lipids [44]. Chlordane (t-nonachlor) (aOR = 4.6; 95% CI, 0.5–41.6) and HCB (aOR = 6.4; 95% CI, 1.0–42.8) showed a similar trend [44]. Aldrin, β-hexachlorocyclohexane (β-BHC) and mirex also had increased ORs; however, few women had concentrations above the limit of detection preventing further analysis. Two other studies yielded similar results. Specifically, hexachlorocyclohexane (HCH) was associated with an increased risk of endometriosis in a large study with 248 surgically confirmed endometriosis cases and 538 controls [45]. β-HCH concentrations were significantly elevated in the serum (third vs. lowest quartile: OR = 1.7; 95% CI: 1.0–2.8; highest vs. lowest quartile OR = 1.3; 95% CI: 0.8–2.4), as well as for mirex (highest vs. lowest category: OR = 1.5; 95% CI: 1.0–2.2). The results were adjusted for participant age, reference date year, serum lipids, education, race/ethnicity, smoking, and alcohol intake. Although trends were seen throughout multiple forms of endometriosis, the strongest association was seen in women with ovarian endometriosis. Similarly, γ-hexachlorocyclohexane (γ-HCH) had a significant association with endometriosis risk (adjusted OR (AOR) for age, body mass index, breast-feeding conditional on parity, cotinine, and lipids = 1.27; 95% CI: 1.01–1.59) [31]. Although these studies provide evidence for a link between exposure to different pesticides and increased risk of endometriosis, there are several limitations to note. In particular, while the authors adjusted their data for some potential confounding variables none appeared to adjust for BMI. Moreover, since multiple pesticides were quantified in each study, correction for multiple comparisons would add confidence to the findings and exclude the potential for type I error. Furthermore, the lack of a dose–response relationship [45] suggests that chance discovery cannot be excluded.

We found no recent animal studies and only one *in vitro* study was found. HCB treatment enhanced MMP-2 and MMP-9 activities in human endometrial stromal cell line T-HESC, primary cultures of Human Uterine Fibroblast (HUF), and ESCs [46]. Specifically, MMP-2 was only elevated in ESCs, whereas MMP-9 was elevated in all models. An increase in COX-2 and prostaglandin receptor-4 expression, prostaglandin E_2 secretion and the c-Src kinase activation in T-HESC was also seen after HCB exposure. The results suggest that HCB may promote inflammation and invasion parameters through regulation of the AhR pathway.

In summary, the epidemiological and biomonitoring studies suggest a potential association between exposure to chlorinated organic pesticides and increased risk of endometriosis; however, study limitations cannot exclude chance discovery owing to multiple comparisons, failure to adequately adjust for important confounders and lack of a dose–response relationship all weaken confidence in the link between COP exposure and endometriosis risk. A single tissue culture animal experiment conducted within the search window suggests that it is biologically plausible for COPs to promote endometriosis risk. Consequently, we suggest weak evidence linking exposure to COPs and endometriosis.

3.3 Perfluoroalkyl and polyfluoroalkyl substances

Perfluoroalkyl substances are a rather unique group of compounds due to their seemingly harmless properties. However, over the last decade, perfluoroalkyl and polyfluoroalkyl substances have been detected in blood and urine across the globe [47, 48]. Compromised of carbon-fluorine atoms, this extremely strong bond forms stable compounds that are used in clothing, cookware, carpets, and other common household items. Exposure to these compounds has been linked to adverse effects on metabolism, immune function, and fertility [49–51].

In a case–control study [27], nine perfluorochemicals (PFCs) were measured in the blood of study participants by liquid chromatography–tandem mass spectrometry. Surgical visualization was used to confirm endometriosis in the operative population and MRI was used to confirm the absence of endometriosis in the control population. Both perfluorooctanoic acid (PFOA; OR = 1.89 [95% CI = 1.17–3.06]) and perfluorononanoic acid (PFNA) (2.20 [1.02–4.75]) were seen to be associated with endometriosis risk, where results were only moderately changed when adjusted for fecundity [27]. Patients with more severe stages of endometriosis (Stages III and IV) showed a higher concentration of perfluorooctane sulfonic acid (1.86 [1.05–3.30]) and PFOA (2.58 [1.18–5.64]) in their blood compared to controls [27]. Although this study shows a significant association between PFC exposure with an apparent dose response, there are a number of limitations to consider. First assignments of healthy study participants to the control population using MRI alone to exclude asymptomatic endometriosis cannot exclude women with endometriosis. Undiagnosed endometriosis was found in 45.3% of asymptomatic women undergoing laparoscopies for benign conditions [1] and thus the potential for misclassification error in this study weakens confidence in the purported association. Finally, circulating concentration of PFCs from the NHANES (2003–2006) study was compared in 753 women with self-reported diagnosis compared to healthy women without a diagnosis of endometriosis [52]. Results from this study showed that PFNA, PFOA, and perfluorooctane sulfonate (PFOS) were significantly higher among women with endometriosis compared to the control population. Women in the referent population of this study were significantly younger, non-Hispanic white, had more than one menstrual period in the last year and reported to be pregnant at the time of the exam. Furthermore, use of self-reported diagnosis of endometriosis may introduce group assignment bias and thus, these data must be interpreted with caution.

The data linking exposure to Perfluoroalkyl substances and endometriosis are limited to the results of two biomonitoring studies. Although the results suggest that women with endometriosis have exposure to Perfluoroalkyl substances, any potential association with endometriosis is weak owing to limitations of these studies and absence of experimental animal studies or mechanistic experiments.

3.4 Bisphenol A (BPA)

A monomeric compound, bisphenol A (BPA) is used to polymerize plastics and can be found in common household items such as toilet paper, water bottles, the lining of tin cans, cash register receipts, dental sealants, and building supplies [53]. With over a million tons of BPA being used in the United States alone, BPA has become ubiquitous in the environment leading to widespread human exposure. BPA is able to bind to both estrogen receptors (Esr1 and Esr2), activate the estrogen signaling cascade and thus is considered a xenoestrogen [54]. Estrogenic capacity has led some to postulate that BPA exposure may play a role in the pathophysiology of endometriosis (**Table 2**).

A population-based case–control study [56], analyzed the urine from 143 women with confirmed or suspected endometriosis (cases) and 287 healthy controls. Urinary creatinine concentrations, age, reference year, as well as both ovarian and non-ovarian pelvic endometriosis were taken into account. Overall, the urinary BPA concentrations in cases did not differ from the control group. However, unconditional logistic regression analysis revealed that the second versus lowest quartile and third versus lowest quartile had increased adjusted odds ratio (aOR 3.0; 95% CI: 1.2–7.3 and aOR 3.0; 95% CI: 1.1–7.6) for higher BPA concentrations in women with non-ovarian pelvic endometriosis; however, there was no association

Authors	Cases vs. controls	Exposure Investigated	Tissue	Outcome
Simonelli et al. [55]	68:60	BPA	Urine and peritoneal fluid	Urinary BPA levels were found in all analyzed samples; with a statistically significant difference between patients and controls. Urinary BPA concentrations were significantly greater (p = 0.001) in women with endometriosis compared to the control group.
Upson et al. [56]	143:287	BPA	Urine	No statistically significant association between total urinary BPA concentrations and endometriosis overall. However, significant results were seen in urine in relation to non-ovarian pelvic endometriosis (2nd quartile vs. lowest quartile: OR = 3.0; 95% CI: 1.2–7.3 and 3rd vs. lowest quartile: OR = 3.0; 95% CI: 1.1–7.6), but not ovarian endometriosis.
Cobellis et al. [57]	58:11	BPA and BPB	Serum	BPA was found in 51.7% and BPB was found in sera 27.6% but either could not be detected in all the control cases. Suggests an association between at least one of the compound endometriosis risk.
Itoh et al. [58]	166 infertile women	BPA	Urine	No significant (p = 0.24) association of endometriosis with urinary BPA concentration.

Table 2.
Summary of exposures and outcomes in epidemiological studies designed to investigate the association between Bisphenol A (BPA) exposure and endometriosis.

between urine BPA concentrations and ovarian endometriosis. Moreover, there was no relationship between the highest urine concentrations of BPA and endometriosis overall as well as for non-ovarian pelvic endometriosis and ovarian endometriosis. Furthermore, the lack of a dose–response relationship with increasing urine concentrations of BPA weakens confidence in the potential link between BPA exposure and endometriosis risk.

Results of biomonitoring studies revealed that mean BPA concentrations in the plasma of infertile women with endometriosis (n = 11), polycystic ovarian syndrome (PCOS, n = 31) and PCOS plus endometriosis (n = 3) combined (4.66 ± 3.52, 95% CI; 3.60–5.72 ng/ml) were significantly greater than in a control population (n = 34) of healthy fertile women (2.64 ± 3.99, 95% CI; 1.24–4.03 ng/ml) [59]. In women who reported a diagnosis of endometriosis, the mean ± (SD) concentration of BPA was 4.59 ± 1.22 ng/ml (range < LOQ – 5.31 ng/ml). Moreover, BPA concentrations were quantifiable in only 3% of study participants and comparisons with the fertile controls was not reported. Given the ubiquitous nature of BPA, the low detection frequency in this study is rather surprising and thus we interpret these findings with caution. The small sample size, self-reported diagnosis of endometriosis and associated potential for misclassification error are important limitations of this study. Results of a much larger cross-sectional study of 166 Japanese women [58], showed no significant difference in BPA levels in the urine. BPA concentrations were non-significantly (p = 0.24) greater in women with endometriosis stage 0–I (median = 0.74 μg/g after adjusting to creatinine levels), whereas women with stages II-IV endometriosis had a median concentration of 0.93 μg/g creatinine [58]. BPA levels measured in the sera from healthy fertile (n = 11) and endometriotic women (n = 58) found that both BPA and bisphenol B (BPB) levels were detectable in 51.7% and 27.6% of cases, respectively whereas the control patients showed a complete absence of both compounds [57]. Recently, urinary concentrations of BPA were significantly greater in women (n = 68) with endometriosis (1.17–12.68 pg/μl) compared to a control population (n = 60) (1.28–2.35 pg/μl) [55]. Finally, BPA has a short half-life and the measures in women with a diagnosis of endometriosis are temporally disconnected from the onset of disease which may have originated years earlier in time. The interval between onset of symptoms and diagnosis ranges from 6 to 12 years [34] and thus exposure measurements made after diagnosis are difficult to link with the development of endometriosis. Therefore, reverse causation cannot be excluded as a potential explanation for differences in circulating concentrations of the toxicants measured.

In an animal study [60], BPA and bisphenol AF (BPAF) affected endometriosis lesion development in ovariectomized and hormonally intact mice specific to dose and hormonal status of the host mouse. Minced uterine tissue was injected into the peritoneal cavity of host mice. In this study, BPA treatment disrupted ovarian steroidogenic pathways resulting in lower progesterone levels and higher atretic oocyte numbers [60]. BPAF and BPA had higher epithelial proliferation scores, although this was only significant in the highest dose of 900 ppm. Both compounds mimicked estrogen, with BPAF having a stronger effect than estrogen [60]. Taken together, these data suggest that BPA and related compounds can affect mechanisms important in the pathophysiology of endometriosis. However, the concentrations of BPA needed to achieve these effects are higher than human exposure and thus are unlikely to be relevant at the concentrations of BPA measured in the general human population in contemporary studies.

Results of a tissue culture experiments demonstrated that BPA treatment arrested human ESCs at the G2/M phase of the cell cycle, allowing for cell migration. Progesterone amplifying receptors such as insulin growth factor binding protein 1 and prolactin were also increased in response to BPA treatment [61]. These results suggest that BPA exposure could modulate endometrial stromal cells function; however, the effective concentrations exceed human exposure. Consequently, ambiguous study results from biomonitoring studies and lack of animal studies suggests a lack of association between BPA exposure and risk of endometriosis.

3.5 Phthalate esters

Phthalate esters are used as a softener in polyvinyl chloride plastics to make plastics flexible and can be found in products such as cosmetics, building materials, and in medical equipment such as intravenous bags, tubing and rubber stoppers in syringes and blood collection tubes. Phthalates leach from finished products leading to ubiquitous human exposure [62, 63]. Exposure to phthalate esters has been linked with decreased circulating testosterone [64] and animal experiments have shown that phthalates are competitive antagonists of the androgen receptor that displace testosterone from the receptor increasing its availability for conversion to estrogens via aromatase [65]. Therefore, it is postulated that exposure to phthalates could be associated with increased risk of endometriosis (**Table 3**).

A large case–control study [67], examined 626 women (495 cases; 131 controls) from 14 clinical centers. Study participants in both groups had a laparoscopy or a pelvic MRI to diagnose the presence of endometriosis. Among the 14 phthalate metabolites, mono-n-butyl phthalate, mono-[(2-carboxymethyl) hexyl] phthalate, mono (2-ethyl-5-carboxyphentyl) phthalate, mono (2-ethylhexyl) phthalate, mono (2-ethyl-5-hydroxyhexyl) phthalate, and mono (2-ethyl-5-oxohexyl), all showed two-fold significant increase in the odds of diagnosis. Results were adjusted for age, BMI, and creatinine. Depending on the method of diagnosis, monooctyl phthalate

Authors	Cases vs. controls	Exposure investigated	Tissue	Outcome
Pednekar et al. [59]	34:45	BPA, MMP, MBzP, MEHP, MEHHP, MiBP-d4 and BPA-d6	Plasma	Significantly higher plasma concentrations of MBzP (95% CI; 11.69–28.12 versus 3.34–8.10), BPA (95% CI; 3.60–5.72 versus 1.24–4.03), and MEHHP (95% CI; 5.10–8.43 versus 0.58–2.85).
Nazir et al. [66]	50: 50	DEHP	Serum	The mean (± SD) DEHP concentration in cases was 65.29 ± 21.69 ng/ml and undetectable in controls. An increasing trend was seen across stages (I-IV).
Buck Louis et al. [67]	495:131	DEHP, mECPP, mCMHP, mEOHP, mEHHP, mEHP, mCPP, mMP, miBP, mBP, mCHP, mBzP, mNP, and mOP,	Urine	MBP, mCMHP, mECPP, mEHP, mEHHP, mEOHP, all showed a two-fold significant increase in the odds of diagnosis.
Huang et al. [68]	28: 29	MBP	Urine	Increase in urinary mono-n-butyl phthalate (94.1 versus 58.0 microg/g creatinine, $p < 0.05$) in women with endometriosis compared to controls.
Itoh et al. (2009)	57:80	MEP, MBP, MBzP, MEHP, mEOHP, and MEHHP	Urine	No significant ($p = 0.23–0.90$) association between endometriosis and any urinary creatinine-adjusted phthalate measured.
Weuve et al. [69]	n = 1227	MEHP, BMP, MEP, and MBzP	Urine	Positive associations for MBP (OR = 1.36; 95% CI, 0.77–2.41) for the highest versus lowest three quartiles, and inverse associations for MEHP in relation to endometriosis (OR = 0.44; 95% CI, 0.19–1.02)
Huang et al. [70]	44:69	MMP, MEP, MnBP, MBzP, MEHP, 5oxo-MEHP, 5OH-MEHP	Urine	Marginally increased level of urinary MEHP only.
Upson et al. [45, 71]	92:195	MEHP, MEHHP, MEOHP, MECPP, MBzP, MEP, MiBP, MnBP	Urine	Greater urinary concentrations of MBzP and MEP in the urine of women with endometriosis compared to controls. Strong inverse association between urinary MEHP and endometriosis risk (aOR 0.3, 95% CI: 0.1–0.7).

Table 3.
Summary of exposures and outcomes in epidemiological studies designed to investigate the association between phthalate exposure and endometriosis.

was restricted to surgical diagnosis of endometriosis with histological confirmation, whereas mono (2-ethylhexyl) phthalate was restricted to surgical diagnosis alone. However potential limitations may arise through adding concentrations as mECPP, mEHHP, mEOHP where all are metabolites of DEHP that were elevated in the operative cohort. Yet when summing DEHP metabolites (mECPP, mCMHP, mEHHP, mEOHP, and mEHP), there is a higher odds of endometriosis in the control population cohort. A further limitation is the lack of adjustment for multiple comparisons and thus chance discovery cannot be excluded. A large study from the National Health and Nutrition Examination Survey (NHANES, 1999–2004), examined phthalate levels in 1227 women, with a self-reported history of endometriosis and uterine leiomyomata. MEHP, monobutyl phthalate (MBP), monoethyl phthalate (MEP), and MBzP levels were measured in patients with each disease as well as patients that reported both [69]. Comparing the highest versus lowest three quartiles of urinary phthalate levels, MBP had an OR of 1.36 (95% CI, 0.77–2.41), MEHP was 0.44 (95% CI, 0.19–1.02), with no association for MEP and MBzP in endometriosis patients. Significantly higher plasma concentration of DBP which is broken down into MBP was also seen [69]. However, the use of self-reported cases may be unreliable. Contrary to the NHANES study, an increased endometriosis risk with an increase in urinary MBzP and MEP was described although the results were not significant [71]. Moreover, an inverse relationship between endometriosis risk and urinary MEHP was found (OR = 0.3; 95% CI = 0.1–0.7) and an inverse relationship was also suggested for DEHP, MEHHP, mono-(2-ethyl-5-oxohexyl) phthalate (MEOHP) and ΣDEHP. Therefore, a compelling link between phthalate exposure and endometriosis has not been established.

Results of several biomonitoring studies have documented higher concentrations of phthalate metabolites in the urine of women with endometriosis compared to a reference population. Plasma concentrations of mono-methyl phthalate (MMP), mono-benzyl phthalate (MBzP), mono-2-ethylhexyl phthalate (MEHP) and mono-(2-ethyl-5-hydroxyhexyl) phthalate (MEHHP) were recently quantified by gas chromatography–mass spectrometry in infertile women with endometriosis (n = 11), polycystic ovarian syndrome (PCOS, n = 31) and PCOS plus endometriosis (n = 3) and 34 fertile women without evidence of gynecological disorders [59]. Overall, the mean (± SD) concentrations (ng/ml) of MBzP (19.9 ± 27.3 95% CI;11.69–28.12) and MEHHP (6.76 ± 5.54, 95% CI; 5.10–8.43) were significantly higher in infertile women compared to fertile women (5.72 ± 6.82, 95% CI; 3.34–8.10 and 1.71 ± 3.24, 0.58–2.85; respectively), whereas no differences were detected between groups for MMP and MEHP. The mean concentrations of MBzP and MEHHP in women with endometriosis were 40.9 ± 51.4 (range < LOQ – 116.5) and 5.43 ± 5.53 ng/ml (range < LOQ – 14.76), respectively. However, only 4–5% of women with endometriosis had concentrations of MBzP and MEHHP above the LOQ. Study participants were assigned to groups based upon self-reports of gynecological diagnoses which is open to misclassification error. In addition, the small sample size overall together with the limited number of study participants with quantifiable concentrations of phthalates are important limitations of this study.

Recently, differences in serum DEHP concentrations were found between women with endometriosis and control patients using high-performance liquid chromatography [66]. The mean ± SD concentration of DEHP in cases (n = 50) was 65.3 ± 21.7 ng/ml, whereas it was undetectable in the controls. Among the four stages of the disease, women with endometriosis showed a linear increase in DEHP concentration with more advanced stages, although the sample size for stage I was n = 1. Age groups did not impact DEHP serum levels. Controversy remains, as DEHP is broken down by glutathione S-transferase and P450 enzyme, which has been reported to be compromised in endometriosis patients [72]. This may explain the difference in serum concentration, as the control patients are able to metabolize DEHP into metabolites which were not recorded. A further weakness of this study is the measurement of DEHP in the serum rather than metabolites in either the serum or urine and thus the potential for sample contamination cannot be discounted.

A group from Taiwan investigated the association between GSTM1 polymorphisms and phthalates in adenomyosis, leiomyoma and endometriosis [68]. Although no relationship between the gene and the disease was found, there was an increase in urinary mono-n-butyl phthalate (94.1 versus 58.0 microg/g creatinine, $p < 0.05$) among the 28 women with endometriosis relative to the 29 controls.

In a subsequent study [70], the potential relationship between polymorphisms of CYP17A1 and phthalate exposure was explored in women with leiomyoma (fibroids, n = 36), endometriosis or adenomyosis (n = 44) and healthy controls (n = 69). However, only a marginally increased level of urinary MEHP was found in patients with endometriosis or adenomyosis [70].

Our search failed to identify any experimental animal studies and only two mechanistic studies were located. MMP-2 and 9 activities, cellular invasiveness, Erk phosphorylation, and p21-activated kinase 4 expression (PAK4) were increased in endometrial stromal cell cultures exposed to DEHP [73]. All five significantly elevated markers play a role in cellular division, actin cytoskeletal dynamics, motility, cell survival, and immune defense [73, 74]. Another study found that DEHP treatment increased ESC reactive oxygen species (ROS) generation and decreased expression of superoxide dismutase (SOD), glutathione peroxidase (GPX), heme oxygenase (HO), and catalase (CAT). p-ERK/p-p38 and NF-κB were also increased [75]. This provides a potential explanation for the decreased expression of antioxidant enzymes and increased ROS. Lastly, Esr1 expression was also increase proportional to dose [75].

In summary, while several studies revealed higher phthalate esters concentrations in women with endometriosis compared to controls the results of epidemiological studies remain equivocal. Moreover, the short half-life of 5–6 h for these chemicals suggests that higher concentrations detected in women with endometriosis compared to controls may be a consequence of the disease rather than a causal factor and thus reverse causation cannot be excluded. While *in vitro* studies suggest that phthalate esters can adversely affect mechanisms relevant to the pathophysiology of endometriosis, the effective concentrations are beyond human exposure and thus are unlikely to be clinically important.

3.6 Metals

Trace metals are nearly impossible to avoid in one's lifetime, as they are found both naturally in our bodies and are produced during industrial processes. Exposure to metals has been reported to interfere with cell proliferation, migration, cell degeneration, oxidative stress, and apoptosis, nearly all of which are properties of endometriosis [76]. Therefore, a link between circulating concentrations of metals and endometriosis has been explored by several groups.

A positive relationship between lead and endometriosis (adjusted OR = 2.59, 95% CI = 1.11–6.06) was found in Asian women whereas zinc levels were inversely associated with the disease (adjusted OR = 0.39, 95% CI = 0.18–0.88) [77]. While cadmium (Cd) levels were greater in women with endometriosis, the adjusted odds ratio was not significant [77]. Furthermore, no significant relationship was found between 20 trace elements quantified in the urine and three in blood [76]. Cases were surgically confirmed, whereas the controls were confirmed for the absence of endometriosis through MRI. Contrary to the findings by [24], Cd was inversely related to endometriosis risk, while urinary chromium and copper were marginally associated with endometriosis (aOR = 1.97; 95% CI: 1.21–3.19; aOR = 2.66; 95% CI: 1.26–5.64) [76]. Comparisons for each of the metals increase the probability of chance discovery and thus any association is considered suspect.

Our search of the literature failed to reveal any recent animal studies; however, a tissue culture study revealed that Cd treatment-induced higher ESC proliferation (p = 0.02) in cultures derived from eutopic endometrium of women with endometriosis compared to controls [78]. Although the mechanism was not identified, it is suggested that Cd at 10^{-5} M is the toxic threshold for ESCs [78], a concentration that is orders of magnitude above typical human exposure.

In summary, biomonitoring studies offer weak support for a potential link between metals exposure and endometriosis. Moreover, results from a tissue culture experiment suggest that Cd can adversely affect ESC proliferation but only at concentrations far in excess of human exposure. Consequently, we consider the evidence of a link between exposure to metals and risk of endometriosis to be speculative at best.

4. Future directions

The current literature fails to provide compelling evidence for an association between exposure to environmental toxicants and endometriosis risk. Although current evidence is weak, involvement of environmental toxicants in the pathophysiology of endometriosis cannot be excluded. However, we propose that establishing a link between exposure to environmental toxicants and endometriosis is particularly challenging. Endometriosis is a heterogeneous disease in which peritoneal and ovarian endometriomas may arise by mechanisms that differ from DIE [79] and thus environmental interactions may be different from other forms of the disease.

Absence of diagnostic tools such as a blood test for endometriosis together with normalization of pelvic pain and use of oral contraceptives among other factors leads to lengthy delays in diagnosis. Importantly, the interval between the onset and symptoms and definitive diagnosis of disease can be lengthy varying between 6 and 12 years [34]. Thus, there is a temporal disconnection between collection of biological samples for analysis and the onset of disease. Hence, the use of case–control studies may not permit convincing evidence of an association and the potential for reverse causation cannot be excluded.

Identification of appropriate control groups poses an additional challenge since the prevalence of endometriosis in asymptomatic women can be high [1]. Furthermore, the hallmarks of endometriosis include chronic pelvic pain and infertility. Women dealing with chronic pain and or infertility may adopt activities or behaviors to reduce their pain or improve their chances of conceiving that diverge from the healthy fertile population and thus their exposures may be a function of disease status rather than factors contributing to the pathophysiology of endometriosis. Consequently, in the absence of clinical tools to diagnosis endometriosis, the most appropriate control group in the future may be symptomatic women undergoing laparoscopy with careful inspection of the pelvic cavity to exclude the presence of endometriosis, even though this step is admittedly imperfect [80].

Epidemiological studies that adjust for potential confounders (e.g. age, BMI, parity, breast feeding, cigarette smoking, and alcohol consumption) and account for multiple comparisons could prove valuable in elucidating the role of exposure to environmental toxicants in the pathophysiology of endometriosis. Finally, it is unlikely that any group of women are exposed to a singly chemical or group of chemicals and thus quantification of chemicals from different chemical groups in a single study with an appropriate control, control for confounds and correction for multiple comparisons could prove informative.

In the absences of robust epidemiological data experimental animal studies take on greater importance for establishing biological plausibility of a potential association. In general, there is a paucity of literature addressing the potential hazards of environmental toxicants in the survival and growth of endometriotic implants in animal models of endometriosis. While spontaneous endometriosis is predominately limited to humans and some non-human primates, animal xenotransplant models using dispersed cells from ectopic implants in women with endometriosis can provide valuable insight into potential chemical hazards relevant to endometriosis and mechanisms. However, dose levels used should include a concentration representative of human exposure. Similarly, tissue culture studies are essential for mechanistic insight; however, we propose that test concentrations should cover a range of doses that include concentrations below and representative of human exposure as well as high doses through to toxic levels.

5. Summary and conclusions

While in general, the epidemiological studies are judged to provide weak evidence of an association between exposure to environmental toxicants and endometriosis, a potential link cannot be excluded. Animal and cell culture models suggest biologically plausible mechanisms between the environmental toxicant exposures and endometriosis risk; however, the effective concentrations exceed human exposure levels. Consequently, we conclude that a causal relationship between exposure to any environmental toxicant and endometriosis does not currently exist, but the evidence does not allow us to exclude a potential link.

Author details

Shay M. Freger and Warren G. Foster*
Department of Obstetrics and Gynecology, McMaster University, Hamilton, Ontario, Canada

*Address all correspondence to: fosterw@mcmaster.ca

References

[1] Rawson JM. Prevalence of endometriosis in asymptomatic women. The Journal of Reproductive Medicine. 1991;**36**:513-515

[2] Sampson J. Peritoneal endometriosis due to the menstrual dissemination of endometrial tissue into the peritoneal cavity. American Journal of Obstetrics and Gynecology. 1927;**14**:422-469

[3] Matta K, Ploteau S, Coumoul X, Koual M, Le Bizec B, Antignac JP. et al. Associations between exposure to organochlorine chemicals and endometriosis in experimental studies: A systematic review protocol. Environment International. 2019;**124**:400-407

[4] Missmer SA, Hankinson SE, Spiegelman D, Barbieri RL, Marshall LM, Hunter DJ. Incidence of laparoscopically confirmed endometriosis by demographic, anthropometric, and lifestyle factors. American Journal of Epidemiology. 2004;**160**:784-796

[5] Upson K, Sathyanarayana S, Scholes D, Holt VL. Early-life factors and endometriosis risk. Fertility and Sterility. 2015;**104**:964.e965-971.e965

[6] Rier SE, Martin DC, Bowman RE, Dmowski WP, Becker JL. Endometriosis in rhesus monkeys (*Macaca mulatta*) following chronic exposure to tetrachlorodibenzo-p-dioxin. Fundamental and Applied Toxicology. 1993;**21**:433-441

[7] Cano-Sancho G, Ploteau S, Matta K, Adoamnei E, Louis GB, Mendiola J, et al. Human epidemiological evidence about the associations between exposure to organochlorine chemicals and endometriosis: Systematic review and meta-analysis. Environment International. 2019;**123**:209-223

[8] Louis GM, Weiner JM, Whitcomb BW, Sperrazza R, Schisterman EF, Lobdell DT, et al. Environmental PCB exposure and risk of endometriosis. Human Reproduction. 2005;**20**:279-285

[9] Porpora MG, Ingelido AM, Domenico AD, Ferro A, Crobu M, Pallante D, et al. Increased levels of polychlorobiphenyls in Italian women with endometriosis. Chemosphere. 2005;**63**(8):1361-1367

[10] Reddy BS, Rozati R, Reddy S, Kodampur S, Reddy P, Reddy R. High plasma concentrations of poly-chlorinated biphenyls and phthalate esters in women with endometriosis: A prospective case control study. Fertility and Sterility. 2006;**85**:775-779

[11] Lebel G, Dodin S, Ayotte P, Marcoux S, Ferron LA, Dewailly E. Organochlorine exposure and the risk of endometriosis. Fertility and Sterility. 1998;**69**:221-228

[12] Pauwels A, Schepens PJC, Hooghe TD, Delbeke L, Dhont M, Brouwer A, et al. The risk if endometriosis and exposure to dioxins and polychlorinated biphenyls: A case-control study of infertile women. Human Reproduction. 2001;**16**:2050-2055

[13] Tsukino H, Hanaoka T, Sasaki H, Motoyama H, Hiroshima M, Tanaka T, et al. Associations between serum levels of selected organochlorine compounds and endometriosis in infertile Japanese women. Environmental Research. 2005;**99**:118-125

[14] Anger DL, Foster WG. The link between environmental toxicant exposure and endometriosis. Frontiers in Bioscience. 2008;**13**:1578-1593

[15] Foster WG, Agarwal SK. Environmental contaminants and dietary factors in endometriosis. Annals of the New York Academy of Sciences. 2002;**955**:213-229

[16] Foster WG. Do environmental contaminants adversely affect human reproductive physiology? Journal of Obstetrics and Gynaecology Canada. 2003;**25**:33-44

[17] Foster WG. Endocrine toxicants including 2,3,7,8-terachlorodibenzo-p-dioxin (TCDD) and dioxin-like chemicals and endometriosis: Is there a link? Journal of Toxicology and Environmental Health. Part B, Critical Reviews. 2008;**11**:177-187

[18] Vabre P, Gatimel N, Moreau J, Gayrard V, Picard-Hagen N, Parinaud J, et al. Environmental pollutants, a possible etiology for premature ovarian insufficiency: A narrative review of animal and human data. Environmental Health. 2017;**16**:37

[19] Faroon O, Ruiz P. Polychlorinated biphenyls: New evidence from the last decade. Toxicology and Industrial Health. 2016;**32**:1825-1847

[20] Bruner-Tran KL, Osteen KG. Dioxin-like PCBs and endometriosis. Systems Biology in Reproductive Medicine. 2010;**56**:132-146

[21] Korach KS, Sarver P, Chae K, McLachlan JA, McKinncy JD. Estrogen receptor-binding activity of poly-chlorinated hydroxybiphenyls: Conformationally restricted structural probes. Molecular Pharmacology. 1988;**33**:120-126

[22] Moore M, Mustain M, Daniel K, Chen I, Safe S, Zacharewski T, et al. Antiestrogenic activity of hydroxylated polychlorinated biphenyl congeners identified in human serum. Toxicology and Applied Pharmacology. 1997;**142**:160-168

[23] Porpora MG, Medda E, Abballe A, Bolli S, De Angelis I, di Domenico A, et al. Endometriosis and organochlorinated environmental pollutants: A case-control study on Italian women of reproductive age. Environmental Health Perspectives. 2009;**117**:1070-1075

[24] Cai LY, Izumi S, Suzuki T, Goya K, Nakamura E, Sugiyama T, et al. Dioxins in ascites and serum of women with endometriosis: A pilot study. Human Reproduction. 2010;**26**(1):117-126

[25] Trabert B, De Roos AJ, Schwartz SM, Peters U, Scholes D, Barr DB, et al. Non-dioxin-like polychlorinated biphenyls and risk of endometriosis. Environmental Health Perspectives. 2010;**118**:1280-1285

[26] Ploteau S, Antignac JP, Volteau C, Marchand P, Vénisseau A, Vacher V, et al. Distribution of persistent organic pollutants in serum, omental, and parietal adipose tissue of French women with deep infiltrating endometriosis and circulating versus stored ratio as new marker of exposure. Environment International. 2016;**97**:125-136

[27] Louis GM, Peterson CM, Chen Z, Hediger ML, Croughan MS, Sundaram R, et al. Perfluorochemicals and endometriosis: The ENDO study. Epidemiology. 2012;**23**:799-805

[28] Martínez-Zamora MA, Mattioli L, Parera J, Abad E, Coloma JL, van Babel B, et al. Increased levels of dioxin-like substances in adipose tissue in patients with deep infiltrating endometriosis. Human Reproduction. 2015;**30**:1059-1068

[29] Simsa P, Mihalyi A, Schoeters G, Koppen G, Kyama CM, Den Hond EM, et al. Increased exposure to dioxin-like compounds is associated with endometriosis in a case-control study in women. Reproductive Biomedicine Online. 2010;**20**:681-688

[30] Vichi S, Medda E, Ingelido AM, Ferro A, Resta S, Porpora MG, et al. Glutathione transferase polymorphisms

and risk of endometriosis associated with polychlorinated biphenyls exposure in Italian women: A gene-environment interaction. Fertility and Sterility. 2012;**97**:1143-1151

[31] Buck Louis GM, Chen Z, Peterson CM, Hediger ML, Croughan MS, Sundaram R, et al. Persistent lipophilic environmental chemicals and endometriosis: The ENDO study. Environmental Health Perspectives. 2012;**120**:811-816

[32] Matsuzaka Y, Kikuti YY, Goya K, Suzuki T, Cai LY, Oka A, et al. Lack of an association human dioxin detoxification gene polymorphisms with endometriosis in Japanese women: Results of a pilot study. Environmental Health and Preventive Medicine. 2012;**17**:512-517

[33] Sinaii N, Cleary SD, Younes N, Ballweg ML, Stratton P. Treatment utilization for endometriosis symptoms: A cross-sectional survey study of lifetime experience. Fertility and Sterility. 2007;**87**:1277-1286

[34] Greene R, Stratton P, Cleary SD, Ballweg ML, Sinaii N. Diagnostic experience among 4,334 women reporting surgically diagnosed endometriosis. Fertility and Sterility. 2009;**91**:32-39

[35] Bruner-Tran KL, Ding T, Osteen KG. Dioxin and endometrial progesterone resistance. Seminars in Reproductive Medicine. 2010;**28**:59-68

[36] Bruner-Tran KL, Rier SE, Eisenberg E, Osteen KG. The potential role of environmental toxins in the pathophysiology of endometriosis. Gynecologic and Obstetric Investigation. 1999;**48**(Suppl 1):45-56

[37] Rier SE, Tuner WE, Martin DC, Morris R, Lucier GW, Clark GC. Serum levels of TCDD and dioxin-like chemicals in rhesus monkeys chronically exposed to dioxin: Correlation of increased serum PCB levels with endometriosis. Toxicological Sciences. 2001;**59**:147-159

[38] Yang JZ, Agarwal SK, Foster WG. Subchronic exposure to 2,3,7,8-tetrachlorodibenzo-p-dioxin modulates the pathophysiology of endometriosis in the Cynomolgus monkey. Toxicological Sciences. 2000;**56**:374-381

[39] Huang Q, Chen Y, Chen Q, Zhang H, Lin Y, Zhu M, et al. Dioxin-like rather than non-dioxin-like PCBs promote the development of endometriosis through stimulation of endocrine-inflammation interactions. Archives of Toxicology. 2017;**91**:1915-1924

[40] Wang Y, Chen H, Wang N, Guo H, Fu Y, Xue S, et al. Combined 17β-estradiol with TCDD promotes M2 polarization of macrophages in the endometriotic milieu with aid of the interaction between endometrial stromal cells and macrophages. PLoS One. 2015;**10**:e0125559

[41] Resuehr D, Glore DR, Taylor HS, Bruner-Tran KL, Osteen KG. Progesterone-dependent regulation of endometrial cannabinoid receptor type 1 (CB1-R) expression is disrupted in women with endometriosis and in isolated stromal cells exposed to 2,3,7,8-tetrachlorodibenzo-p-dioxin (TCDD). Fertility and Sterility. 2012;**98**:948.e941-956.e941

[42] Willing C, Peich M, Danescu A, Kehlen A, Fowler PA, Hombach-KlonischS.Estrogen-independent actions of environmentally relevant AHR-agonists in human endometrial epithelial cells. Molecular Human Reproduction. 2011;**17**:115-126

[43] Hu T, Yao M, Fu X, Chen C, Wu R. Polychlorinated biphenyl 104 promotes migration of endometrial

stromal cells in endometriosis. Toxicology Letters. 2018;**290**:19-28

[44] Cooney MA, Buck Louis GM, Hediger ML, Vexler A, Kostyniak PJ. Organochlorine pesticides and endometriosis. Reproductive Toxicology. 2010;**30**:365-369

[45] Upson K, De Roos AJ, Thompson ML, Sathyanarayana S, Scholes D, Barr DB, et al. Organochlorine pesticides and risk of endometriosis: Findings from a population-based case-control study. Environmental Health Perspectives. 2013;**121**:1319-1324

[46] Chiappini F, Bastón JI, Vaccarezza A, Singla JJ, Pontillo C, Miret N, et al. Enhanced cyclooxygenase-2 expression levels and metalloproteinase 2 and 9 activation by hexachlorobenzene in human endometrial stromal cells. Biochemical Pharmacology. 2016;**109**:91-104

[47] Calafat AM, Kuklenyik Z, Caudill SP, Reidy JA, Needham LL. Perfluorochemicals in pooled serum samples from United States residents in 2001 and 2002. Environmental Science & Technology. 2006;**40**:2128-2134

[48] Guruge KS, Taniyasu S, Yamashita N, Wijeratna S, Mohotti KM, Seneviratne HR, et al. Perfluorinated organic compounds in human blood serum and seminal plasma: A study of urban and rural tea worker populations in Sri Lanka. Journal of Environmental Monitoring. 2005;**7**:371-377

[49] Bach CC, Vested A, Jørgensen KT, Bonde JP, Henriksen TB, Toft G. Perfluoroalkyl and polyfluoroalkyl substances and measures of human fertility: A systematic review. Critical Reviews in Toxicology. 2016;**46**:735-755

[50] Kielsen K, Shamim Z, Ryder LP, Nielsen F, Grandjean P, Budtz-Jørgensen E, et al. Antibody response to booster vaccination with tetanus and diphtheria in adults exposed to perfluorinated alkylates. Journal of Immunotoxicology. 2016;**13**:270-273

[51] Liu G, Dhana K, Furtado JD, Rood J, Zong G, Liang L, et al. Perfluoroalkyl substances and changes in body weight and resting metabolic rate in response to weight-loss diets: A prospective study. PLoS Medicine. 2018;**15**:e1002502

[52] Campbell S, Raza M, Pollack AZ. Perfluoroalkyl substances and endometriosis in us women in NHANES 2003-2006. Reproductive Toxicology. 2016;**65**:230-235

[53] Rashtian J, Chavkin DE, Merhi Z. Water and soil pollution as determinant of water and food quality/contamination and its impact on female fertility. Reproductive Biology and Endocrinology. 2019;**17**:5

[54] Rochester JR. Bisphenol a and human health: A review of the literature. Reproductive Toxicology. 2013;**42**:132-155

[55] Itoh H, Iwasaki M, Hanaoka T, Sasaki H, Tanaka T, Tsugane S. Urinary phthalate monoesters and endometriosis in infertile Japanese women. Science of the Total Environment. 2009;408:37-42

[56] Upson K, Sathyanarayana S, De Roos AJ, Koch HM, Scholes D, Holt VL. A population-based case-control study of urinary bisphenol A concentrations and risk of endometriosis. Human Reproduction. 2014;**29**:2457-2464

[57] Cobellis L, Colacurci N, Trabucco E, Carpentiero C, Grumetto L. Measurement of bisphenol A and bisphenol B levels in human blood sera from healthy and endometriotic women. Biomedical Chromatography. 2009;**23**:1186-1190

[58] Itoh H, Iwasaki M, Hanaoka T, Sasaki H, Tanaka T, Tsugane S. Urinary

bisphenol-A concentration in infertile Japanese women and its association with endometriosis: A cross-sectional study. Environmental Health and Preventive Medicine. 2007;**12**:258-264

[59] Pednekar PP, Gajbhiye RK, Patil AD, Surve SV, Datar AG, Balsarkar GD, et al. Estimation of plasma levels of bisphenol-A & phthalates in fertile & infertile women by gas chromatography-mass spectrometry. The Indian Journal of Medical Research. 2018;**148**:734-742

[60] Jones RL, Lang SA, Kendziorski JA, Greene AD, Burns KA. Use of a mouse model of experimentally induced endometriosis to evaluate and compare the effects of bisphenol A and bisphenol AF exposure. Environmental Health Perspectives. 2018;**126**:127004

[61] Forte M, Mita L, Cobellis L, Merafina V, Specchio R, Rossi S, et al. Triclosan and bisphenol A affect decidualization of human endometrial stromal cells. Molecular and Cellular Endocrinology. 2016;**422**:74-83

[62] Silva MJ, Barr DB, Reidy JA, Malek NA, Hodge CC, Caudill SP, et al. Urinary levels of seven phthalate metabolites in the U.S. population from the national health and nutrition examination survey (NHANES) 1999-2000. Environmental Health Perspectives. 2004;**112**:331-338

[63] Tyrrell J, Melzer D, Henley W, Galloway TS, Osborne NJ. Associations between socioeconomic status and environmental toxicant concentrations in adults in the USA: NHANES 2001-2010. Environment International. 2013;**59**:328-335

[64] Meeker JD, Ferguson KK. Urinary phthalate metabolites are associated with decreased serum testosterone in men, women, and children from NHANES 2011-2012. The Journal of Clinical Endocrinology and Metabolism. 2014;**99**(11):4346-4352

[65] Lague E, Tremblay JJ. Antagonistic effects of testosterone and the endocrine disruptor mono-(2-ethylhexyl) phthalate on INSL3 transcription in Leydig cells. Endocrinology. 2008;**149**:4688-4694

[66] Nazir S, Usman Z, Imran M, Lone KP, Ahmad G. Women diagnosed with endometriosis show high serum levels of diethyl hexyl phthalate. Journal of Human Reproductive Sciences. 2018;**11**:131-136

[67] Buck Louis GM, Peterson CM, Chen Z, Croughan M, Sundaram R, Stanford J, et al. Bisphenol A and phthalates and endometriosis: The endometriosis: Natural history, diagnosis and outcomes study. Fertility and Sterility. 2013;**100**:162-169

[68] Huang PC, Tsai EM, Li WF, Liao PC, Chung MC, Wang YH, et al. Association between phthalate exposure and glutathione S-transferase M1 polymorphism in adenomyosis, leiomyoma and endometriosis. Human Reproduction. 2010;**25**:986-994

[69] Weuve J, Hauser R, Calafat AM, Missmer SA, Wise LA. Association of exposure to phthalates with endometriosis and uterine leiomyomata: Findings from NHANES, 1999-2004. Environmental Health Perspectives. 2010;**118**:825-832

[70] Huang PC, Li WF, Liao PC, Sun CW, Tsai EM, Wang SL. Risk for estrogen-dependent diseases in relation to phthalate exposure and polymorphisms of CYP17A1 and estrogen receptor genes. Environmental Science and Pollution Research International. 2014;**21**:13964-13973

[71] Upson K, Sathyanarayana S, De Roos AJ, Thompson ML, Scholes D, Dills R, et al. Phthalates and risk of endometriosis. Environmental Research. 2013;**126**:91-97

[72] Kubiszeski EH, de Medeiros SF, da Silva Seidel JA, Barbosa JS, Galera MF, Galera BB. Glutathione s-transferase M1 and T1 gene polymorphisms in Brazilian women with endometriosis. Journal of Assisted Reproduction and Genetics. 2015;**32**:1531-1535

[73] Kim SH, Cho S, Ihm HJ, Oh YS, Heo SH, Chun S, et al. Possible role of phthalate in the pathogenesis of endometriosis: In vitro, animal, and human data. The Journal of Clinical Endocrinology and Metabolism. 2015;**100**:E1502-E1511

[74] Dart AE, Wells CM. P21-activated kinase 4—Not just one of the PAK. European Journal of Cell Biology. 2013;**92**:129-138

[75] Cho YJ, Park SB, Han M. Di-(2-ethylhexyl)-phthalate induces oxidative stress in human endometrial stromal cells in vitro. Molecular and Cellular Endocrinology. 2015;**407**:9-17

[76] Pollack AZ, Louis GM, Chen Z, Peterson CM, Sundaram R, Croughan MS, et al. Trace elements and endometriosis: The ENDO study. Reproductive Toxicology. 2013;**42**:41-48

[77] Lai GL, Yeh CC, Yeh CY, Chen RY, Fu CL, Chen CH, et al. Decreased zinc and increased lead blood levels are associated with endometriosis in Asian women. Reproductive Toxicology. 2017;**74**:77-84

[78] Silva N, Tennekoon K, Senanayake H, Samarakoon S. Metalloestrogen cadmium stimulates proliferation of stromal cells derived from the eutopic endometrium of women with endometriosis. Taiwanese Journal of Obstetrics & Gynecology. 2013;**52**:540-545

[79] Gordts S, Koninckx P, Brosens I. Pathogenesis of deep endometriosis. Fertility and Sterility. 2017;**108**:872.e871-885.e871

[80] Wykes CB, Clark TJ, Khan KS. Accuracy of laparoscopy in the diagnosis of endometriosis: A systematic quantitative review. BJOG. 2004;**111**:1204-1212

Chapter 2

Endocrine Disrupting Chemicals in Cosmetics and Personal Care Products and Risk of Endometriosis

Francisco M. Peinado, Luz M. Iribarne-Durán,
Olga Ocón-Hernández, Nicolás Olea
and Francisco Artacho-Cordón

Abstract

In the last years, the variety and consumption of cosmetics and personal care products (PCPs) have greatly increased, although the long-term adverse effects to low doses of chemicals used in their production and with proven hormone-mimicking properties have been still poorly addressed. Among these endocrine disrupting chemicals (EDCs), parabens, benzophenones, bisphenols, and phthalates are the most widely found in these products. Given the estrogenic-dependent nature of the endometrium, it has been hypothesized the potential contribution of these EDCs contained in cosmetics and PCPs in the risk of endometriosis. In this book chapter, we have summarized the current evidence supporting this hypothesis, highlighting epidemiological, *in vivo,* and *in vitro* studies that have addressed the potential influence of parabens, benzophenones, bisphenols, and phthalates in the origin and progression of this chronic feminine disease.

Keywords: cosmetics, personal care products, endometriosis, endocrine disruptors

1. Introduction

The term "cosmetic" has its origin from the Greek term "kosme'tikos," a noun to denote the art of beautifying the body [1]. Since ancient times, humans have searched for materials and developed many products to mainly enhance female beauty. Over the centuries, cosmetics have been developed and influenced by different ethnic traditions, from the times of the Pharaohs to the modern times [2]. Since then, physical appearance has been an inseparable part of daily human existence, improving their self-image and self-esteem. However, the esthetic concept of beauty has changed overtime, and beauty standards have been modified according to many factors such as social, ethnic, and religious belief influences [2]. Personal hygiene has been also part of human life since the ancient times. Traditionally related to hygiene habits during religious activities, the preparation of food, or the

IntechOpen

Use	Products
Baby care products	Shampoo, lotion, oil, cream, talcum powder
Eyes	Eyebrow and eyeliner pencils, eye shadow, eye make-up remover, lash mascara
Skin care	Blush, powder, make-up base, make-up corrector, cream, lotions, face mask, face cleaner, skin toner, moisturizers
Lips	Lipstick, lip gloss, lip balm, lip liner
Hygiene	Soap, powder, oil, bath salts, shampoo, cleaning wipes
Deodorants and antiperspirants	Deodorants, antiperspirants
Hair	Hair dye, shampoo, coloured shampoo, hair spray, hair conditioner, hair lightener, permanent wave, hair straightener, hair lotion, hair wax
Nails	Base coat, nail polish, cuticle softener, nail polish remover, nail oil, nail glitter
Mouth	Toothpaste, mouthwash
Shaving	Shave balm, lotion, shaving cream/foam, soap
Tanning / UV protection	Oil, cream, sunscreen, suntan lotion
Hair removal	Depilatory wax/cream, oil
Skin lightening	Lightening cream
Feminine hygiene	Pads, panty liners, tampons, wipes, bactericidal creams and solutions

Table 1.
Most used cosmetics and personal care products.

prevention of diseases, hygiene practices have also greatly changed through the cultures and eras, from bathing facilities in the Roman period to modern synthetic products such as body lotions or hair tonics [3].

In the last years, the variety of cosmetics and personal care products (PCPs) have greatly increased (**Table 1**), in parallel to their manufacturing and consumption volumes in developed and developing countries. For example, the consumption of cosmetics and perfumery in Spain has consecutively increased in the last years, reaching a total of 1280 million units sold of these products and 770 million units exported during 2018. To date, the USA is the leader in the consumption of cosmetics and perfumery, with an amount of 78.6 billion euros, followed by China (52 billion euros), Japan (32 billion euros), and Brazil (28 billion euros) [4]. Despite the current beauty standards are not similar along cultures and ethnicities, it is acknowledged that women have a greater use of cosmetics and personal care products (PCPs) when compared with men [5], and therefore, potential adverse effect may affect predominantly to this population.

Table 1 summarizes the main types of cosmetics and PCPs commonly used worldwide.

2. Endocrine disruptors in cosmetics and PCPs

2.1 What is an endocrine disruptor?

The World Health Organization defines an endocrine disrupting chemical (EDC) as an exogenous substance or mixture of substances that alter one or more functions of the endocrine system and consequently cause adverse effects on the health of an intact organism or its progeny [6].

The main characteristics of exposure to EDCs are as follows [7–10]:

- There is no safe dose of EDCs. They act at low concentrations and in combination with endogenous hormones, making it difficult to establish a threshold level of no effect.

- Exposure to EDCs during periods of special vulnerability of the individual's development—pregnancy, lactation, puberty—causes damage with adverse effects throughout their lives and descendants.

- The curves that relate the exposure doses to EDCs with the adverse effect are not linear. The response does not always increase in the same proportion as the exposure dose.

- In general terms, individuals are not exposed to a single type of EDC but to a mixture of EDCs. Therefore, the effects are difficult to predict given the possible synergistic, additive, or antagonistic actions between chemical residues (the cocktail effect).

- As a result of exposure to EDCs in a certain individual, consequences can be observed in subsequent generations, due to either genomic involvement or epigenetic mechanisms. There is great difficulty in establishing a causal association because the effects observed after exposure can occur after long latency periods.

2.2 Sources and routes of exposure to EDCs

EDCs are distributed in the environment due to their widespread use. Depending on their resistance to physical, chemical, and biological degradation as well as their degree of liposolubility, EDCs can be divided into "persistent EDCs" and "non-persistent EDCs." In the case of persistent EDCs, low biodegradability, volatility, bioaccumulation in the trophic chain, and biomagnification are its most outstanding characteristics [11]. Furthermore, they can be transmitted to the offspring through the mother during pregnancy and lactation [12]. Since the 1970s, most countries have banned or severely restricted the production, handling, and disposal of the majority of them due to consistent evidence of their adverse effects at doses traditionally considered safe [13, 14]. Despite this, global population is suspected to be primarily exposed to these pollutants through diet, given the bioaccumulation pattern of these chemicals in the food chain [14].

On the other hand, non-persistent EDCs are less liposoluble, and therefore, they are prone to be metabolized and excreted rapidly [15, 16]. In addition to a variety of pesticides such as glyphosate or permethrins, this group includes bisphenol-A (BPA) and its analogues, parabens (PBs) [methyl- (MeP), ethyl- (EtP), propyl- (PrP), and butyl-paraben (BuP)], phthalates, and benzophenones (BPs). Currently, there is diverse evidence showing the presence of numerous EDC families (mainly phthalates, bisphenols, parabens, and benzophenones) in cosmetic products and PCPs [17–20]. However, contrary to most persistent EDCs, international regulation of their production, handling, and disposal is limited to a reduction in the concentrations of some specific compounds for those cosmetics in the EU market (EU 1004/2014). **Table 2** summarized the trade name, CAS number, and hormonal activity attributed to some of the most frequently used EDCs in cosmetics and PCPs.

Phthalates are used as a plasticizer in cosmetics and PCPs. The study carried out by Gao and Kannan [17] recently revealed that phthalates were found in >90% of the 77 feminine hygiene products analyzed. Mainly, they were found in all the tested pads, panty liners, tampons, and wipes. Furthermore, phthalates were also found in bactericidal creams and solutions, deodorant sprays, and powders. In another study, Guo and Kannan [18] showed that phthalates were also present in leave-on products, such as skin lotions, hair care products, perfumes, skin toners, deodorants, and creams. In this regard, detectable levels of phthalates were found in face creams, eyeliner creams, hand creams, sunscreens, lipsticks, and nail polish. These EDCs were also detected in products for dental hygiene and rinse-off

Compound	Acronym	CAS	Hormonal activities		
			Estrogenic	Anti-androgenic	Thyroid disruption
Bis(2-ethylhexyl) phthalate	DEHP	117-81-7		X	X
Diisononyl phthalate	DiNP	28553-12-0		X	
Dibutyl phthalate	DBP	84-74-2		X	
Diisobutyl phthalate	DiBP	84-69-5		X	
Benzyl butyl phthalate	BBP	85-68-7		X	
Dipentyl phthalate	DPP	131-18-0		X	
Di-n-hexyl Phthalate	DnHP	84-75-3		X	X
Di-n-octyl phthalate	DnOP	117-84-0		X	X
Bisphenol-A	BPA	80-05-7	X		
Methyl-paraben	MeP	99-76-3	X		
Ethyl-paraben	EtP	120-47-8	X		
Propyl-paraben	PrP	94-13-3	X		
Butyl-paraben	BuP	94-26-8	X		
Benzophenone-1	BP-1	131-56-6	X		
Benzophenone-3	BP-3	131-57-7	X		
Octamethylcyclotetrasiloxane	D4	556-67-2	X		
Ethylhexyl 4-methoxycinnamate	EHMC	5466-77-3	X		X
Bencilidene camphor	3-BC	15087-24-8			

Trade name, CAS number and demonstrated hormonal activities.

Table 2.
Most common endocrine disrupting chemicals in cosmetics and personal care products.

products (including body wash, shampoos, hair conditioners, face cleaners, and shaving gels).

In the case of the PB family, its main use in cosmetic products and PCPs is due to their antimicrobial properties [21]. It has been shown that the use of mixtures of paraben congeners allows the increase of their preservative capacity with the use of lower levels of each compounds [19]. Average daily application rates per women for face creams, hand or body lotions, facial cleansers, shampoos, and bath gel were 2.1, 8.7, 4.1, 12.8, and 14.5 g, respectively [22]. Yazar and Johnsson [20] carried out a study where they verified the composition of a series of 204 cosmetic products, which included shampoos, hair conditioners, liquid soap, wipes from different brands, and stores. The results showed that at least 44% of the analyzed cosmetics contained at least one PB congener. The PB that was found in the highest proportion was MeP (41% of the products), followed by PrP (25%). In the study carried out by Gao and Kannan [17], it was found that all feminine hygiene products contained at least one PB, and both MeP and EtP were found in >80% of these compounds, mainly in wipes, creams, bactericide solutions, deodorant sprays, and powders. Moreover, it has been reported that PBs were detected in 40% of the dental hygiene products analyzed and 60% in other types of daily hygiene products. MeP and PrP were the most detected compounds (40% of the analyzed samples), followed by BuP (~20%). The highest concentrations of MeP, EtP, PrP, and BuP ranged between 1040 and 8200 μg/g, which represent approximately 0.1–0.8% per product by weight [18]. Another study carried out in China [19] found PBs in all the categories of PCPs analyzed. Almost all creams, lotions, and face cleaners contained MeP and PrP, with concentrations of MeP slightly higher than PrP (2830 and 1560 μg/g, respectively). Their presence was greater in creams and lotions than in shampoos and body soaps.

BPs are used as ultraviolet (UV) filters. As shown in the study carried out by Rastogi [23], 75 sunscreen products from Europe and the USA tested contained levels of up to three UV filters. A recent study [24] verified the presence of BP-1 and BP-3 in 19.1% of their analyzed products (283 samples analyzed), especially in makeup products, which represented 45.2% of the products with the presence of BPs.

In addition to these three families, the chemical composition of cosmetics and PCPs also contains many other compounds, although with a lower percentage of the presence in these products. Among them, bisphenols, camphenes, dimethicones, and oxycinnamates can be found. Within these minority families, bisphenols are the one that are usually found in the greatest presence in cosmetic products. The main use of BPA is the manufacture of epoxy resins, obtaining polycarbonate plastics, which have great mechanical and thermal stability, as well as very good transparency [25], while the main use of the families of camphenes, dimethicones, and oxycinnamates is that they are used as preservatives in the manufacture of PCPs [26, 27]. Nevertheless, the concentrations of these substances in cosmetics and PCPs have been poorly addressed.

Contrary to persistent EDCs that mainly reach body internal compartments through diet, the main route of human exposure to non-persistent EDCs released from cosmetics and PCPs is mainly the dermal route [28]. Therefore, these EDCs avoid the first-pass metabolism, enhancing the bioavailability and therefore the biological effect of the parent compounds [15]. In this regard, several studies have related to the use of cosmetics and PCPs and internal levels of PB and BPs. For example, it has been recently found that levels of some PB and BPs in menstrual blood are related to the use of cosmetics [29]. Moreover, urinary concentrations of PBs were related to the use of hair products, deodorants, face, and hand creams [30]. Similarly, Larsson et al. [31] found higher levels of PBs and phthalates among those women with higher use of hygiene products.

2.3 Mechanisms of action of EDCs

EDCs act at very different levels of complexity, interfering a variety of hormone-signaling pathways. For instance, they can modify the circulating levels of hormones by acting on their synthesis, metabolism, or degradation. They can also reduce, increase, or interfere with the specific receptors for hormonal action and therefore affect the ability to respond to natural hormones [32]. In the particular case of EDCs that interfere in steroid hormone-related signaling pathways, the observed effects seem to be linked to the activation/blocking of nuclear receptors, which are the most common modes of action responsible for dose curves with non-monotonic response in experimental studies [33]. In fact, many EDCs released from cosmetics and PCPs have been evidenced to exert estrogenic and antiandrogenic activities in both *in vivo* and *in vitro* studies [34–40] (see **Table 2**).

An increasing number of studies have also linked exposure to EDCs with epigenetic changes in humans [41, 42]. An unexposed individual may show epigenetic changes due to (1) altered ovum or sperm after EDC exposure or (2) in utero exposure to EDCs. In this regard, it has been evidenced that fetal exposure to environmental pollutants with endocrine disrupting properties such as mirex, chlordane, or *p,p´*-DDE can cause epigenetic changes with transgenerational effects [43, 44]. This is also the case of bisphenol-A (BPA), and PBs, with epigenetic changes after prenatal and adolescence exposures to these chemicals [45, 46].

Furthermore, inflammation and oxidative stress have also been recently postulated as possible mechanisms of action of EDCs [47–50]. In this regard, oxidative stress, that is, the imbalance between the production of free radicals and the antioxidant capacity, has been shown to be enhanced after exposure to a variety of EDCs, including PBs and BPs [47, 49, 50]. For instance, human exposure to PB and BP has been linked to higher levels of lipid peroxidation [50, 51]. Moreover, local disruption of the antioxidant capacity has also been reported [47]. Although the underlying mechanisms are still poorly understood, it has been suggested that, at least in part, EDCs might induce oxidative stress via estrogen receptor-α signaling pathways [52]. Moreover, EDC exposure has also been evidenced to trigger an inflammatory microenvironment [50, 53]. With an intimate relationship, both oxidative and inflammatory responses have also been suggested as crucial mechanisms beyond a variety of chronic diseases, as well as some gynecological conditions such as endometriosis [54, 55].

3. Potential adverse effects of EDC exposure

The consequences of exposure to EDCs seem to be different depending on age and gender (**Table 3**). In the case of men, EDC exposure is suspected to cause alterations in the development of the genitourinary system including cryptorchidism, testicular cancer, and infertility [56, 57]. Among women, the increase in hormone-dependent cancers (either breast or ovarian) [56] as well as uterine fibroids and endometriosis might also be related to inadvertent exposure to EDCs. Moreover, chronic conditions such as metabolic syndrome and its components (obesity, insulin resistance, hypertension, or dyslipidemia), neurobehavioral development disorders, and poor thyroid function are also on the list of possible effects of EDC exposure. In particular, in utero exposure to EDCs is believed to have consequences of such magnitude that they would hardly be suspected in studies of adult individuals. For example, in utero exposure to some EDCs has been linked to increased risk for breast cancer or endometriosis [58, 59]. This association gives maternal exposure some very particular peculiarities and places women of childbearing age in the limelight of most studies on endocrine disruption.

3.1 Use of cosmetics and PCPs and feminine diseases

Over the years and in parallel with the change in people's habits and lifestyle, numerous evidence has revealed that cosmetics could cause a variety of disease conditions in humans. For instance, women are suspected to have a greater risk for some chronic conditions such as obesity and metabolic syndrome than men [60], and in addition to physiological differences between genders, the greater female consumption of cosmetics and PCPs might also underlie this enhanced risk. Moreover, the consumption of cosmetics and PCPs might also be beyond the development of female-specific diseases such as breast or ovarian cancer. In this regard, Darbre [61]

Women	Girls	Boys	Men	Women / Men
Endometriosis	Precocious puberty	Cryptorchidism and hypospadias	Testicular cancer	Obesity
Breast / vaginal / ovarian / endometrial cancer	Early breast and pubic hair development	Reduction in semen quality	Prostate cancer	Diabetes
Uterine fibroids	Congenital malformations	Reduction in testosterone levels	Reduction in semen quality	Elevated blood pressure
Gestational diabetes and pregnancy-related outcomes	Low birth weight	Low birth weight	Reduction in testosterone levels	Dyslipidemia
Impaired ovarian function	Cognitive impairments	Cognitive impairments		
Polycystic ovary syndrome				
Reduced fertility				

Table 3.
Some adverse effects of EDCs in humans.

first alarmed scientific community about the potential effect of PCPs in breast cancer, suggesting that underarm cosmetic use might increase breast cancer. In fact, they detected a variety of EDCs including PBs in breast tumors, with higher concentrations in those samples from the axilla region, suggesting that their concentrations might be related to the application of deodorant products, body lotions, sprays, moisturizers, and sunscreen products in areas close to the human breast. However, current evidence on the relationship between cosmetic/PCP use and risk of cancer is not very conclusive. In this regard, in a case-control study comprised by 209 cases of breast cancer and 209 healthy controls, Linhart and Talasz [62] reported that the greater use of underarm cosmetic products was associated with increased risk of breast cancer. Contrary, a cohort study did not found any association between use of skincare products and risk of cancer of the breast and endometrium [63]. Another study carried out by McGrath [64] reported that those women with a higher use of antiperspirant products were diagnosed with breast cancer at an earlier age. Furthermore, it has been observed that long-term exposure to body care creams containing ethinyl estradiol may increase the risk of abnormal genital bleeding and breast cancer [65]. Interestingly, a case-report study found that synthetic hormones found in lotions used by the mother were present in very high concentrations in the hair of the girl [66].

However, the variety of products and differences in dosage, patterns of use, and individual susceptibility to specific product formulations pose great difficulties to detect a potential effect of cosmetic and PCP habits on human adverse effects [36, 61, 67–69]. Thus, the use of internal burden of EDCs seems to better reflect the magnitude of cosmetic and PCP use, independently of the type of product used or the dose applied. In this regard, urinary levels of PBs have been related to greater risk for breast cancer [70]. Some studies have also addressed the potential association between exposure to PCP-released EDCs and the origin and development of other female diseases. In this regard, the presence of trace levels of PBs was found in endometrial tissue samples suspected of being related to an increased risk of endometrial carcinoma [71]. Levels of PrP were also related to diminished ovarian reserve in a prospective cohort study of the US women seeking fertility treatment [72]. Regarding the development of sex characteristics during puberty, a recent study observed associations between levels of PBs and earlier development of the breasts and the pubic hair in girls. Moreover, earlier menarche was also related to higher levels of PBs [73].

Regarding BPs, *in vitro* studies have shown that exposure to BPs in rats and mice has been related to feminized sexual behavior and increased uterine weight [39, 74]. Two *in vivo* studies have also demonstrated the disturbance caused by BP in ovarian tissue [75, 76]. Santamaría and Abud [75] found that exposure to BP-1 and BP-3 disrupted early events in ovarian cells, such as germ cell development and disruption of crucial gene expression related to follicular assembly. Similarly, Shin and Go [76] reported the induction of BP-dependent metastasis in an *in vivo* model for ovarian cancer. Moreover, an epidemiological study has reported that urinary BP levels might be associated with blood pressure during pregnancy [77]. Similarly, higher BP levels were related to thyroid hormones and growth factors in pregnant women, as well as to reduced fetal growth [74].

Other hormonally active chemicals widely used in cosmetics are phthalates. Exposure to various congeners has been associated with the appearance of various female diseases. Exposure to di-(2-ethylhexyl) phthalate has been linked to an increased risk of preterm delivery [78–80] and intrauterine growth restriction [81]. Furthermore, it has also been associated with reduced total oocyte yield and a reduced probability of achieving pregnancy and live birth [82]. Other phthalate congeners, such as monoethyl phthalate and dibutyl phthalate, have also been linked to decreased fertility in women [79, 83].

Several investigations have also suggested the potential association between BPA exposure and adverse outcomes in women. For instance, it has been shown that elevated serum or urine BPA levels are associated with anovulation [84], lower antral follicle counts [85, 86], preterm birth [87], and infertility [88]. Moreover, increasing urinary BPA levels were associated with delayed menarche in adolescent girls [89, 90]. Furthermore, higher BPA levels have been associated with an increased risk of developing polycystic ovary syndrome [84, 91–93], ovarian failure [94], infertility [95], and fibroids [96, 97]. Triclosan, widely present in soaps, detergents, and toothpaste, has also been related to decreased fertility [98], although the currently available evidence is scarce.

3.2 Associations between PCP- and cosmetic-released EDCs and endometriosis

As mentioned above, detectable levels of PBs and BPs have been detected in endometrial tissue and menstrual blood [29, 71]. Trace levels of intact PBs were predominantly detected in endometrial carcinoma tissues (23%) in contrast to normal endometrium samples (2%), and thus, authors suggested that they might be related to an increased risk of endometrial carcinoma [71]. On the other hand, several PBs and BPs have been detected in menstrual blood samples, a biological sample in intimate contact with the endometrium [29]. Moreover, these menstrual blood concentrations of PBs and BPs were related to the magnitude of use of creams and cosmetics, evidencing that these EDCs from cosmetics and PCPs are capable of reaching a wide variety of biological matrices and thus might orchestrate, or at least contribute, to the development and progression of multiple gynecological diseases such as endometrial cancer and endometriosis.

Concerning endometriosis, the origin of endometriosis still remains unclear. To date, although various theories have been postulated to give a possible explanation for the origin of endometriosis [99–105], none of them consistently explains the onset and progression of the disease in deeper stages. Currently, it is known that it is a multifactorial disease in which genetic, epigenetic, immunological, hormonal, and environmental factors are involved [106]. Due to the suspected increase in the number of cases in the last decades [107], it is suspected that, in addition to the increased awareness among doctors and patients, environmental risk factors are suspected to also contribute to the onset and progression of this disease. This environmental hypothesis of the origin of the disease is also reinforced due to the estrogen-dependent nature of this pathology [53, 108].

Despite the growing public concern about human risks derived from the use of PCPs and cosmetics, there is little evidence on their influence on endometriosis (**Table 4**). To our knowledge, only one study has investigated the relationship between EDCs released from sunscreens and endometriosis. Concentrations of 2-hydroxy-4-methoxybenzophenone, 2,4-dihydroxybenzophenone, 2,2′-dihydroxy-4-methoxybenzophenone, 2,2′,4,4′-tetrahydroxybenzophenone, and 4-hydroxi-benzophenone were analyzed in urine samples collected from 600 women. The results obtained suggest that exposure to elevated levels of 2,4-dihydroxybenzophenone (BP-3) may be associated with a higher probability of a diagnosis of endometriosis [109]. As authors mentioned, these findings denoted an approximate 65% increase in the odds of an endometriosis diagnosis in women with the highest BP-3 concentration compared to women with lower concentrations.

Regarding BPA exposure, a recent meta-analysis revealed limited and contradictory epidemiological evidence regarding the contribution of BPA in the risk for endometriosis [110]. Thus, despite few studies have reported an absence of association between urinary levels of BPA and disease [111, 112], others reported increased risk for endometriosis [53, 113–115]. Even more, it has been recently suggested that

Ref.	EDCs	Study design	Matrix for exposure assessment	Population	Reported associations
109	Benzophenone (BP-1, BP-2, BP-3, BP-8, 4-OH-BP)	Epidemiological (cohort) ENDO study	Urine	N=600 Operative cohort: 473 Population cohort: 127	↑ urinary BP-3 levels → ↑ endometriosis risk
53	Bisphenol (BPA, BPS, BPF)	Epidemiological (case-control) EndEA study	Urine	N=124: 35 cases and 89 controls	↑ urinary BPA levels → ↑ endometriosis risk
111	Bisphenol (BPA)	Epidemiological (cohort) ENDO study	Urine	N=600 Operative cohort: 473 Population cohort: 127	No association
112	Bisphenol (BPA)	Epidemiological (cross-sectional)	Urine	N=140 women suspected of infertility	No association
114	Bisphenol (BPA)	Epidemiological (case-control)	Urine	N=430: 143 cases and 287 controls	↑ urinary BPA levels → ↑ non-ovarian pelvic endometriosis
115	Bisphenol (BPA)	Epidemiological (case-control)	Urine	N=100: 50 cases and 50 controls	↑ urinary BPA levels → ↑ endometriosis risk
113	Bisphenol (BPA)	Epidemiological (case-control)	Urinary and peritoneal fluid	N=128: 68 cases and 60 controls	↑ urinary BPA levels → ↑ endometriosis risk
116	Bisphenol (BPA)	*In vivo* study	-	136 mice	↑ urinary BPA levels → ↑ endometriosis risk
117	Bisphenol (BPA)	*In vivo* study	-	20 mice	↑ urinary BPA levels → ↑ endometriosis risk
108	Bisphenol (BPA, BPAF)	*In vivo* study	-	185 mice	↑ urinary BPA levels → ↑ atretic oocyte number
118	Phthalates (dBP, bBP, DEHP, dnOP)	Epidemiological (case-control)	Plasma	N=220: 85 cases and 135 controls	↑ urinary phthalate levels → ↑ endometriosis risk
111	Phthalates (mECPP, mCMHP, mEOHP, mEHHP, mEHP, mCPP, mMP, mEP, miBP, mBP, mCHP, mBzP, mNP, mOP)	Epidemiological (cohort) ENDO study	Urine	N=600 Operative cohort: 473 Population cohort: 127	↑ urinary phthalate levels → ↑ endometriosis risk
119	Phthalates (mEHHP, mEOHP, mBP, mBzP, mECPP)	Epidemiological (case-control)	Urine	N=88: 55 cases and 33 controls	↑ urinary phthalate levels → ↑ endometriosis risk
120	Phthalates (mEHP, mBP, mEP, mBzP)	Epidemiological (cross-sectional)	Urine	N=1227: 87 cases of endometriosis, 151 women with uterine fibroids and 1020 healthy women	No association
121	Phthalates (mEHP, mEHHP, mEOHP, mECPP, mBzP, mEP, miBP, mBP)	Epidemiological (case-control)	Urine	N= 287: 92 cases and 195 controls	No association
122	Phthalates (mMP, miBP, mBP, mCHP, mNP, mOP, mBzP, mEHP)	Epidemiological (case-control)	Urine	N= 52: 30 cases and 22 controls	No association

Benophenone-1 (BP-1), benzophenone-2 (BP-2), benzophenone-3 (BP-3), benzophenone-8 (BP-8), 4-hydroxybenzophenone (4-OH-BP), bisphenol A (BPA, bisphenol S (BPS), bisphenol F (BPF), bisphenol AF (BPAF), mono (2-ethyl-5-carboxyphentyl) phthalate (mECPP), mono-[(2-carboxymethyl) hexyl] phthalate (mCMHP), mono (2-ethyl-5-oxohexyl) phthalate (mEOHP), mono (2-ethyl-5-hydroxyhexyl) phthalate (mEHHP), mono (2-ethylhexyl) phthalate (mEHP), mono (3-carboxypropyl) phthalate (mCPP), monomethyl phthalate (mMP), monoethyl phthalate (mEP), mono (2-isobutyl phthalate) (miBP), mono-n-butyl phthalate (mBP), mono-iso-butyl phthalate (miBP), monocyclohexyl phthalate (mCHP), monobenzyl phthalate (mBzP), monoisonoyl phthalate (mNP), and monooctyl phthalate (mOP), dibutyl phthalate (dBP), butyl benzyl phthalate (bBP), di-n-octyl phthalate (dnOP)

Table 4.
Studies exploring associations between exposure to cosmetics- and PCPs-released EDCs and endometriosis.

levels of oxidative stress might act as a mediation effect on the association between exposure to bisphenols and endometriosis risk [53]. Furthermore, exposure to BPA has not only been related to the onset of endometriosis, but it might be also involved in the progression of the disease [112, 114]. Moreover, these findings are supported by different experimental studies. In this sense, recent *in vivo* studies have evidenced in mouse models that exposure to bisphenols in adulthood was related to an increase in the growth of endometrial lesions and the number of atretic oocytes, the interruption of the ovarian steroidogenic pathway, an increase in periglandular fibrosis, and the upregulation of matrix remodeling enzymes [108, 116]. Another *in vivo* study revealed that prenatal exposure to BPA and other bisphenols caused a phenotype similar to endometriosis [117]. These experimental studies suggest that exposure to BPA could be related to the development and progression of endometriosis.

Other EDCs found in cosmetics and PCPs are phthalates. Several studies have explored the existing associations between exposure to these chemicals and endometriosis, showing conflicting results. One of the very first investigations reported higher concentrations of phthalates in women with a confirmed diagnosis of endometriosis [118]. Similarly, two studies evidenced an increased risk of endometriosis in women with higher levels of mono (2-ethylhexyl) phthalate [111, 119]. Conversely, few studies did not found any association between levels of urinary levels of any phthalate congener and enhanced risk for endometriosis [112, 120–122].

Currently, there are no studies that have explored the possible contribution of other EDCs released from cosmetics and PCPs (such as parabens, oxycinnamates, camphenes, and dimethicones) and the risk of endometriosis. Moreover, the combined effect of EDCs released from these products on endometriosis has not been addressed yet.

4. Conclusions

To date, there is still very limited evidence on the potential role of EDCs released from cosmetics and PCPs on the origin and development of endometriosis. In general terms, *in vitro*, *in vivo,* and epidemiological evidence is consistent with the endocrine-disrupting hypothesis set out in this chapter, indicating that EDCs might be in the causal pathway that leads to endometriosis. Nevertheless, in all published studies, the particular effect of specific EDCs was measured, without taking into account the possible synergistic or antagonistic effect that these chemicals can exert when they are present in a mixture. Thus, because its diagnosis is difficult and its treatment is mainly symptomatic, it is vitally necessary to establish preventive measures to avoid as far as possible the origin of this disease. Therefore, it is necessary to carry out well-conducted studies, with appropriate sample size and in which the "gold-standard" diagnosis serves to distinguish between cases and controls. Moreover, the combined effect of multiple EDCs on endometriosis should be addressed. These studies are needed to fully elucidate the potential disrupting properties of these PCP-released EDCs in the gynecological tissues. In this way, preventive measures could be established, the chemical composition of PCPs could be modified by other substances that are not endocrine disruptors, or the use of these cosmetics could be reduced as far as possible.

Acknowledgements

This work was supported by a grant from the Spanish Ministry of Health-FEDER (FIS PI17/01743) and the Research Chair "Antonio Chamorro/Alejandro Otero." It was also partly supported by the European Union Commission (the European Human Biomonitoring Initiative H2020-EJP-HBM4EU) and the Spanish Consortium for Research on Epidemiology and Public Health (CIBERESP). The authors are also grateful to the Carlos III Institute of Health (ISCIII) for the predoctoral research contracts (IFI18/00052 and FI17/00316) granted to F.M. Peinado and L.M. Iribarne-Durán, respectively, and the José María Segovia de Arana contract granted to N. Olea (INT18/00060).

Conflict of interest

The authors declare no conflict of interest.

Author details

Francisco M. Peinado[1†], Luz M. Iribarne-Durán[1†], Olga Ocón-Hernández[1,2], Nicolás Olea[1,3,4,5] and Francisco Artacho-Cordón[1,3,4*]

1 Biohealth Research Institute in Granada (ibs.GRANADA), Granada, Spain

2 Obstetrics and Gynecology Service, San Cecilio University Hospital, Granada, Spain

3 Radiology and Physical Medicine Department, University of Granada, Granada, Spain

4 CIBER Epidemiology and Public Health (CIBERESP), Madrid, Spain

5 Nuclear Medicine Unit, "San Cecilio" University Hospital, Granada, Spain

*Address all correspondence to: fartacho@ugr.es

† These authors equally contributed to this work.

References

[1] Merriam-Webster M. Merriam-Webster's Ninth New Collegiate Dictionary. Vol. 294. Spring Field; 1991

[2] Oumeish O. The cultural and philosophical concepts of cosmetics in beauty and art through the medical history of mankind. Clinics in Dermatology. 2001;**19**:375-386

[3] Smith VS. Clean: A History of Personal Hygiene and Purity. United States: Oxford University Press; 2007

[4] Asociación Nacional de Perfumería y Cosmética: Stanpa. Available from: https://www.stanpa.com/sector-en-cifras/mercado-cosmetico-ue/cosmetica-union-europea/

[5] Biesterbos JW, Dudzina T, Delmaar CJ, Bakker MI, Russel FG, von Goetz N, et al. Usage patterns of personal care products: Important factors for exposure assessment. Food and Chemical Toxicology: An International Journal Published for the British Industrial Biological Research Association. 2013;**55**:8-17

[6] Damstra T, Barlow S, Bergman A, Kavlock R, Kraak G. Global Assessment of the State-of-Science of Endocrine Disruptors 2002.

[7] Anway MD, Skinner MK. Epigenetic transgenerational actions of endocrine disruptors. Endocrinology. 2006;**147** (6 Suppl):S43-S49

[8] Kortenkamp A, Faust M, Scholze M, Backhaus T. Low-level exposure to multiple chemicals: reason for human health concerns? Environmental Health Perspectives. 2007;**115**(Suppl 1):106-114

[9] Skinner MK, Guerrero-Bosagna C. Environmental signals and transgenerational epigenetics. Epigenomics. 2009;**1**(1):111-117

[10] Soto AM, Silvia RM, Sonnenschein C. A plasma-borne specific inhibitor of the proliferation of human estrogen-sensitive breast tumor cells (estrocolyone-I). The Journal of Steroid Biochemistry and Molecular Biology. 1992;**43**(7):703-712

[11] Arrebola JP, Fernández MF, Martín-Olmedo P, Molina-Molina JM, Sánchez-Pérez MJ, Sánchez-Cantalejo E, et al. Adipose tissue concentrations of persistent organic pollutants and total cancer risk in an adult cohort from Southern Spain: Preliminary data from year 9 of the follow-up. The Science of the Total Environment. 2014;**500-501**:243-249

[12] Botella B, Crespo J, Rivas A, Cerrillo I, Olea-Serrano MF, Olea N. Exposure of women to organochlorine pesticides in southern Spain. Environmental Research. 2004;**96**(1): 34-40

[13] Olea N, Fernández M, Martin-Olmedo P. Endocrine disrupters. The case of oestrogenic xenobiotics. Revista de Salud Ambiental. 2001;**1**:6-11

[14] Porta M, Puigdomènech E, Ballester F, Selva J, Ribas-Fitó N, Llop S, et al. Monitoring concentrations of persistent organic pollutants in the general population: The international experience. Environment International. 2008;**34**(4):546-561

[15] Søeborg T, Frederiksen H, Andersson AM. Considerations for estimating daily intake values of nonpersistent environmental endocrine disruptors based on urinary biomonitoring data. Reproduction (Cambridge, England). 2014;**147**(4):455-463

[16] Frederiksen H, Skakkebaek NE, Andersson AM. Metabolism of phthalates in humans. Molecular Nutrition & Food Research. 2007;**51**(7):899-911

[17] Gao CJ, Kannan K. Phthalates, bisphenols, parabens, and triclocarban in feminine hygiene products from the United States and their implications for human exposure. Environment International. 2020;**136**:105465

[18] Guo Y, Kannan K. A survey of phthalates and parabens in personal care products from the United States and its implications for human exposure. Environmental Science & Technology. 2013;**47**(24):14442-14449

[19] Guo Y, Wang L, Kannan K. Phthalates and parabens in personal care products from China: Concentrations and human exposure. Archives of Environmental Contamination and Toxicology. 2014;**66**(1):113-119

[20] Yazar K, Johnsson S, Lind ML, Boman A, Lidén C. Preservatives and fragrances in selected consumer-available cosmetics and detergents. Contact Dermatitis. 2011;**64**(5):265-272

[21] Daniel JW. Metabolic aspects of antioxidants and preservatives. Xenobiotica. 1986;**16**(10-11):1073-1078

[22] United States Environmental Protection Agency (USEPA). Exposure Factors Handbook, 2011. Available from: https://www.epa.gov/expobox/exposure-factors-handbook-chapter-17.

[23] Rastogi SC. UV filters in sunscreen products—a survey. Contact Dermatitis. 2002;**46**(6):348-351

[24] Panico A, Serio F, Bagordo F, Grassi T, Idolo A, Deg M, et al. Skin safety and health prevention: An overview of chemicals in cosmetic products. Journal of Preventive Medicine and Hygiene. 2019;**60**(1):E50-Ee7

[25] Vandenberg LN, Hauser R, Marcus M, Olea N, Welshons WV. Human exposure to bisphenol A (BPA). Reproductive Toxicology. 2007;**24**(2):139-177

[26] Luna-Bastante L, Gatica-Ortega ME, Pastor-NietoMA,Vergara-de-la-CampaL, Gómez-Dorado BA, Alonso-Naranjo L, et al. Allergic contact dermatitis to Tinosorb S, Scutellaria baicalensis, and other emerging allergens in cosmetics. Contact Dermatitis. 2020;**82**(5):307-309

[27] Santonocito M, Salerno B, Trombini C, Tonini F, Pintado-Herrera MG, Martínez-Rodríguez G, et al. Stress under the sun: Effects of exposure to low concentrations of UV-filter 4-methylbenzylidene camphor (4-MBC) in a marine bivalve filter feeder, the Manila clam Ruditapes philippinarum. Aquatic Toxicology. 2020;**221**:105418

[28] Nicolopoulou-Stamati P, Hens L, Sasco AJ. Cosmetics as endocrine disruptors: Are they a health risk? Reviews in Endocrine & Metabolic Disorders. 2015;**16**(4):373-383

[29] Iribarne-Durán LM, Domingo-Piñar S, Peinado FM, Vela-Soria F, Jiménez-Díaz I, Barranco E, et al. Menstrual blood concentrations of parabens and benzophenones and related factors in a sample of Spanish women: An exploratory study. Environmental Research. 2020;**183**:109228

[30] Sakhi AK, Sabaredzovic A, Papadopoulou E, Cequier E, Thomsen C. Levels, variability and determinants of environmental phenols in pairs of Norwegian mothers and children. Environment International. 2018;**114**:242-251

[31] Larsson K, Ljung Björklund K, Palm B, Wennberg M, Kaj L, Lindh CH, et al. Exposure determinants of phthalates, parabens, bisphenol A and triclosan in Swedish mothers and their children. Environment International. 2014;**73**:323-333

[32] Kelce WR, Stone CR, Laws SC, Gray LE, Kemppainen JA, Wilson EM. Persistent DDT metabolite p,p'-DDE is a potent androgen receptor antagonist. Nature. 1995;**375**(6532):581-585

[33] Cookman CJ, Belcher SM. Classical nuclear hormone receptor activity as a mediator of complex concentration response relationships for endocrine active compounds. Current Opinion in Pharmacology. 2014;**19**:112-119

[34] Charles AK, Darbre PD. Combinations of parabens at concentrations measured in human breast tissue can increase proliferation of MCF-7 human breast cancer cells. Journal of Applied Toxicology. 2013;**33**(5):390-398

[35] Chen J, Ahn KC, Gee NA, Gee SJ, Hammock BD, Lasley BL. Antiandrogenic properties of parabens and other phenolic containing small molecules in personal care products. Toxicology and Applied Pharmacology. 2007;**221**(3):278-284

[36] Darbre PD, Harvey PW. Paraben esters: Review of recent studies of endocrine toxicity, absorption, esterase and human exposure, and discussion of potential human health risks. Journal of Applied Toxicology: JAT. 2008;**28**(5):561-578

[37] Kerdivel G, Le Guevel R, Habauzit D, Brion F, Ait-Aissa S, Pakdel F. Estrogenic potency of benzophenone UV filters in breast cancer cells: Proliferative and transcriptional activity substantiated by docking analysis. PLoS One. 2013;**8**(4):e60567

[38] Oishi S. Effects of propyl paraben on the male reproductive system. Food and Chemical Toxicology. 2002;**40**(12):1807-1813

[39] Schlumpf M, Kypke K, Wittassek M, Angerer J, Mascher H, Mascher D, et al. Exposure patterns of UV filters, fragrances, parabens, phthalates, organochlor pesticides, PBDEs, and PCBs in human milk: Correlation of UV filters with use of cosmetics. Chemosphere. 2010;**81**(10):1171-1183

[40] Suzuki T, Kitamura S, Khota R, Sugihara K, Fujimoto N, Ohta S. Estrogenic and antiandrogenic activities of 17 benzophenone derivatives used as UV stabilizers and sunscreens. Toxicology and Applied Pharmacology. 2005;**203**(1):9-17

[41] Collotta M, Bertazzi PA, Bollati V. Epigenetics and pesticides. Toxicology. 2013;**307**:35-41

[42] Perera F, Herbstman J. Prenatal environmental exposures, epigenetics, and disease. Reproductive Toxicology. 2011;**31**(3):363-373

[43] Titus-Ernstoff L, Troisi R, Hatch EE, Hyer M, Wise LA, Palmer JR, et al. Offspring of women exposed in utero to diethylstilbestrol (DES): a preliminary report of benign and malignant pathology in the third generation. Epidemiology (Cambridge, Mass.). 2008;**19**(2):251-257

[44] Titus-Ernstoff L, Troisi R, Hatch EE, Wise LA, Palmer J, Hyer M, et al. Menstrual and reproductive characteristics of women whose mothers were exposed in utero to diethylstilbestrol (DES). International Journal of Epidemiology. 2006;**35**(4):862-868

[45] Goodrich JM, Dolinoy DC, Sánchez BN, Zhang Z, Meeker JD, Mercado-Garcia A, et al. Adolescent epigenetic profiles and environmental exposures from early life through peri-adolescence. Environmental Epigenetics. 2016;**2**(3):dvw018

[46] Park CJ, Nah WH, Lee JE, Oh YS, Gye MC. Butyl paraben-induced changes in DNA methylation in rat epididymal spermatozoa. Andrologia. 2012;**44**(Suppl 1):187-193

[47] Artacho-Cordón F, Ríos-Arrabal S, León J, Frederiksen H, Sáenz JM, Martín-Olmedo P, et al. Adipose tissue concentrations of non-persistent

environmental phenols and local redox balance in adults from Southern Spain. Environment International. 2019;**133** (Pt A):105118

[48] Mustafa M, Garg N, Banerjee BD, Sharma T, Tyagi V, Dar SA, et al. Inflammatory-mediated pathway in association with organochlorine pesticides levels in the etiology of idiopathic preterm birth. Reproductive Toxicology. 2015;**57**:111-120

[49] Thompson PA, Khatami M, Baglole CJ, Sun J, Harris SA, Moon EY, et al. Environmental immune disruptors, inflammation and cancer risk. Carcinogenesis. 2015;**36**(Suppl 1): S232-S253

[50] Watkins DJ, Ferguson KK, Anzalota Del Toro LV, Alshawabkeh AN, Cordero JF, Meeker JD. Associations between urinary phenol and paraben concentrations and markers of oxidative stress and inflammation among pregnant women in Puerto Rico. International Journal of Hygiene and Environmental Health. 2015;**218**(2):212-219

[51] Kang S, Kim S, Park J, Kim HJ, Lee J, Choi G, et al. Urinary paraben concentrations among pregnant women and their matching newborn infants of Korea, and the association with oxidative stress biomarkers. The Science of the Total Environment. 2013;**461-462**:214-221

[52] Cho YJ, Park SB, Park JW, Oh SR, Han M. Bisphenol A modulates inflammation and proliferation pathway in human endometrial stromal cells by inducing oxidative stress. Reproductive Toxicology. 2018;**81**:41-49

[53] Peinado FM, Lendínez I, Sotelo R, Iribarne-Durán LM, Fernández-Parra J, Vela-Soria F, et al. Association of urinary levels of bisphenols A, F, and S with endometriosis risk: Preliminary results of the EndEA study. International Journal of Environmental Research and Public Health. 2020;**17**(4):e1194

[54] Gupta S, Agarwal A, Krajcir N, Alvarez JG. Role of oxidative stress in endometriosis. Reproductive Biomedicine Online. 2006;**13**(1):126-134

[55] Lambrinoudaki IV, Augoulea A, Christodoulakos GE, Economou EV, Kaparos G, Kontoravdis A, et al. Measurable serum markers of oxidative stress response in women with endometriosis. Fertility and Sterility. 2009;**91**(1):46-50

[56] Ibarluzea Jm J, Fernández MF, Santa-Marina L, Olea-Serrano MF, Rivas AM, Aurrekoetxea JJ, et al. Breast cancer risk and the combined effect of environmental estrogens. Cancer Causes & Control. 2004;**15**(6):591-600

[57] Olea N, Fernandez MF. Chemicals in the environment and human male fertility. Occupational and Environmental Medicine. 2007;**64**(7): 430-431

[58] Benagiano G, Brosens I. In utero exposure and endometriosis. The Journal of Maternal-Fetal and Neonatal Medicine. 2014;**27**(3):303-308

[59] Cohn BA, La Merrill M, Krigbaum NY, Yeh G, Park JS, Zimmermann L, et al. DDT exposure in utero and breast cancer. The Journal of Clinical Endocrinology and Metabolism. 2015;**100**(8):2865-2872

[60] Pucci G, Alcidi R, Tap L, Battista F, Mattace-Raso F, Schillaci G. Sex- and gender-related prevalence, cardiovascular risk and therapeutic approach in metabolic syndrome: A review of the literature. Pharmacological Research. 2017;**120**:34-42

[61] Darbre PD. Underarm cosmetics are a cause of breast cancer. European Journal of Cancer Prevention. 2001;**10**(5):389-393

[62] Linhart C, Talasz H, Morandi EM, Exley C, Lindner HH, Taucher S, et al. Use of underarm cosmetic products in relation to risk of breast cancer: A case-control study. eBioMedicine. 2017;**21**:79-85

[63] Rylander C, Veierød MB, Weiderpass E, Lund E, Sandanger TM. Use of skincare products and risk of cancer of the breast and endometrium: A prospective cohort study. Environmental Health: A Global Access Science Source. 2019;**18**(1):105

[64] McGrath KG. An earlier age of breast cancer diagnosis related to more frequent use of antiperspirants/deodorants and underarm shaving. European Journal of Cancer Prevention. 2003;**12**(6):479-485

[65] Komori S, Ito Y, Nakamura Y, Aoki M, Takashi T, Kinuta T, et al. A long-term user of cosmetic cream containing estrogen developed breast cancer and endometrial hyperplasia. Menopause (New York, NY). 2008;**15**(6):1191-1192

[66] Guarneri MP, Brambilla G, Loizzo A, Colombo I, Chiumello G. Estrogen exposure in a child from hair lotion used by her mother: Clinical and hair analysis data. Clinical Toxicology (Philadelphia, PA). 2008;**46**(8):762-764

[67] Darbre PD. Underarm cosmetics and breast cancer. Journal of Applied Toxicology: JAT. 2003;**23**(2):89-95

[68] Darbre PD. Environmental oestrogens, cosmetics and breast cancer. Best Practice & Research. Clinical Endocrinology & Metabolism. 2006;**20**(1):121-143

[69] Harvey PW, Darbre P. Endocrine disrupters and human health: Could oestrogenic chemicals in body care cosmetics adversely affect breast cancer incidence in women? Journal of Applied Toxicology: JAT. 2004;**24**(3):167-176

[70] Parada H Jr, Gammon MD, Ettore HL, Chen J, Calafat AM, Neugut AI, et al. Urinary concentrations of environmental phenols and their associations with breast cancer incidence and mortality following breast cancer. Environment International. 2019;**130**:104890

[71] Dogan S, Tongur T, Erkaymaz T, Erdogan G, Unal B, Sik B, et al. Traces of intact paraben molecules in endometrial carcinoma. Environmental Science and Pollution Research International. 2019;**26**(30):31158-31165

[72] Smith KW, Souter I, Dimitriadis I, Ehrlich S, Williams PL, Calafat AM, et al. Urinary paraben concentrations and ovarian aging among women from a fertility center. Environmental Health Perspectives. 2013;**121**(11-s12):1299-1305

[73] Harley KG, Berger KP, Kogut K, Parra K, Lustig RH, Greenspan LC, et al. Association of phthalates, parabens and phenols found in personal care products with pubertal timing in girls and boys. Human Reproduction (Oxford, England). 2019;**34**(1):109-117

[74] Krause M, Klit A, Blomberg Jensen M, Søeborg T, Frederiksen H, Schlumpf M, et al. Sunscreens: Are they beneficial for health? An overview of endocrine disrupting properties of UV-filters. International Journal of Andrology. 2012;**35**(3):424-436

[75] Santamaría CG, Abud JE, Porporato MM, Meyer N, Zenclussen AC, Kass L, et al. The UV filter benzophenone 3, alters early follicular assembly in rat whole ovary cultures. Toxicology Letters. 2019;**303**:48-54

[76] Shin S, Go RE, Kim CW, Hwang KA, Nam KH, Choi KC. Effect of benzophenone-1 and octylphenol on the regulation of epithelial-mesenchymal transition via an estrogen

receptor-dependent pathway in estrogen receptor expressing ovarian cancer cells. Food and Chemical Toxicology. 2016;**93**:58-65

[77] Liu H, Li J, Xia W, Zhang B, Peng Y, Li Y, et al. Blood pressure changes during pregnancy in relation to urinary paraben, triclosan and benzophenone concentrations: A repeated measures study. Environment International. 2019;**122**:185-192

[78] Ferguson KK, McElrath TF, Ko YA, Mukherjee B, Meeker JD. Variability in urinary phthalate metabolite levels across pregnancy and sensitive windows of exposure for the risk of preterm birth. Environment International. 2014;**70**:118-124

[79] Ferguson KK, McElrath TF, Meeker JD. Environmental phthalate exposure and preterm birth. JAMA Pediatrics. 2014;**168**(1):61-67

[80] Ferguson KK, O'Neill MS, Meeker JD. Environmental contaminant exposures and preterm birth: A comprehensive review. Journal of Toxicology and Environmental Health, Part B: Critical Reviews. 2013;**16**(2):69-113

[81] Zhao Y, Chen L, Li LX, Xie CM, Li D, Shi HJ, et al. Gender-specific relationship between prenatal exposure to phthalates and intrauterine growth restriction. Pediatric Research. 2014;**76**(4):401-408

[82] Hauser R, Gaskins AJ, Souter I, Smith KW, Dodge LE, Ehrlich S, et al. Urinary phthalate metabolite concentrations and reproductive outcomes among women undergoing in vitro fertilization: Results from the EARTH study. Environmental Health Perspectives. 2016;**124**(6):831-839

[83] Kay VR, Chambers C, Foster WG. Reproductive and developmental effects of phthalate diesters in females. Critical Reviews in Toxicology. 2013;**43**(3):200-219

[84] Costa EM, Spritzer PM, Hohl A, Bachega TA. Effects of endocrine disruptors in the development of the female reproductive tract. Arquivos Brasileiros de Endocrinologia e Metabologia. 2014;**58**(2):153-161

[85] Ziv-Gal A, Flaws JA. Evidence for bisphenol A-induced female infertility: A review (2007-2016). Fertility and Sterility. 2016;**106**(4):827-856

[86] Souter I, Smith KW, Dimitriadis I, Ehrlich S, Williams PL, Calafat AM, et al. The association of bisphenol-A urinary concentrations with antral follicle counts and other measures of ovarian reserve in women undergoing infertility treatments. Reproductive Toxicology. 2013;**42**:224-231

[87] Peretz J, Vrooman L, Ricke WA, Hunt PA, Ehrlich S, Hauser R, et al. Bisphenol A and reproductive health: Update of experimental and human evidence, 2007-2013. Environmental Health Perspectives. 2014;**122**(8):775-786

[88] Weinberger B, Vetrano AM, Archer FE, Marcella SW, Buckley B, Wartenberg D, et al. Effects of maternal exposure to phthalates and bisphenol A during pregnancy on gestational age. The Journal of Maternal-Fetal and Neonatal Medicine. 2014;**27**(4):323-327

[89] McGuinn LA, Ghazarian AA, Joseph Su L, Ellison GL. Urinary bisphenol A and age at menarche among adolescent girls: Evidence from NHANES 2003-2010. Environmental Research. 2015;**136**:381-386

[90] Berger K, Eskenazi B, Kogut K, Parra K, Lustig RH, Greenspan LC, et al. Association of prenatal urinary concentrations of phthalates and bisphenol A and pubertal timing in boys and girls. Environmental Health Perspectives. 2018;**126**(9):97004

[91] Palioura E, Diamanti-Kandarakis E. Polycystic ovary syndrome (PCOS) and endocrine disrupting chemicals (EDCs). Reviews in Endocrine & Metabolic Disorders. 2015;**16**(4):365-371

[92] Rutkowska AZ, Diamanti-Kandarakis E. Polycystic ovary syndrome and environmental toxins. Fertility and Sterility. 2016;**106**(4):948-958

[93] Wang Y, Zhu Q, Dang X, He Y, Li X, Sun Y. Local effect of bisphenol A on the estradiol synthesis of ovarian granulosa cells from PCOS. Gynecological Endocrinology. 2017;**33**(1):21-25

[94] Özel Ş, Tokmak A, Aykut O, Aktulay A, Hançerlioğulları N, Engin UY. Serum levels of phthalates and bisphenol-Ain patients with primary ovarian insufficiency. Gynecological Endocrinology. 2019;**35**(4):364-367

[95] Wang B, Zhou W, Zhu W, Chen L, Wang W, Tian Y, et al. Associations of female exposure to bisphenol a with fecundability: Evidence from a preconception cohort study. Environment International. 2018;**117**:139-145

[96] Pollack AZ, Buck Louis GM, Chen Z, Sun L, Trabert B, Guo Y, et al. Bisphenol A, benzophenone-type ultraviolet filters, and phthalates in relation to uterine leiomyoma. Environmental Research. 2015;**137**:101-107

[97] Shen Y, Xu Q, Ren M, Feng X, Cai Y, Gao Y. Measurement of phenolic environmental estrogens in women with uterine leiomyoma. PLoS One. 2013;**8**(11):e79838

[98] Vélez MP, Arbuckle TE, Fraser WD. Female exposure to phenols and phthalates and time to pregnancy: the Maternal-Infant Research on Environmental Chemicals (MIREC) Study. Fertility and Sterility. 2015;**103**(4):1011-20.e2

[99] Starzinski-Powitz A, Zeitvogel A, Schreiner A, Baumann R. Endometriosis--a stem cell disease? Zentralblatt für Gynäkologie. 2003;**125**(7-8):235-238

[100] Sampson JA. Peritoneal endometriosis due to the menstrual dissemination of endometrial tissue into the peritoneal cavity. American Journal of Obstetrics and Gynecology. 1927;**14**:422-469

[101] Mechsner S, Weichbrodt M, Riedlinger WFJ, Bartley J, Kaufmann AM, Schneider A, et al. Estrogen and progestogen receptor positive endometriotic lesions and disseminated cells in pelvic sentinel lymph nodes of patients with deep infiltrating rectovaginal endometriosis: A pilot study. Human Reproduction. 2008;**23**(10):2202-2209

[102] Levander G, Normann P. The pathogenesis of endometriosis; an experimental study. Acta Obstetricia et Gynecologica Scandinavica. 1955;**34**(4):366-398

[103] Koninckx PR, Barlow D, Kennedy S. Implantation versus infiltration: The Sampson versus the endometriotic disease theory. Gynecologic and Obstetric Investigation. 1999;**47**:3-9

[104] Gargett CE. Stem cells in gynaecology. The Australian and New Zealand Journal of Obstetrics and Gynaecology. 2004;**44**(5):380-386

[105] Ferguson BR, Bennington JL, Haber SL. Histochemistry of mucosubstances and histology of mixed müllerian pelvic lymph node glandular inclusions. Evidence for histogenesis by müllerian metaplasia of coelomic epithelium. Obstetrics and Gynecology. 1969;**33**(5):617-625

[106] Vercellini P, Viganò P, Somigliana E, Fedele L. Endometriosis: Pathogenesis

and treatment. Nature Reviews. Endocrinology. 2014;**10**(5):261-275

[107] Eisenberg VH, Weil C, Chodick G, Shalev V. Epidemiology of endometriosis: A large population-based database study from a healthcare provider with 2 million members. BJOG: An International Journal of Obstetrics and Gynaecology. 2018;**125**(1):55-62

[108] Jones RL, Lang SA, Kendziorski JA, Greene AD, Burns KA. Use of a mouse model of experimentally induced endometriosis to evaluate and compare the effects of bisphenol A and bisphenol AF exposure. Environmental Health Perspectives. 2018;**126**(12):127004

[109] Kunisue T, Chen Z, Buck Louis GM, Sundaram R, Hediger ML, Sun L, et al. Urinary concentrations of benzophenone-type UV filters in U.S. women and their association with endometriosis. Environmental Science & Technology. 2012;**46**(8):4624-4632

[110] Wen X, Xiong Y, Qu X, Jin L, Zhou C, Zhang M, et al. The risk of endometriosis after exposure to endocrine-disrupting chemicals: A meta-analysis of 30 epidemiology studies. Gynecological Endocrinology. 2019;**35**(8):645-650

[111] Buck Louis GM, Peterson CM, Chen Z, Croughan M, Sundaram R, Stanford J, et al. Bisphenol A and phthalates and endometriosis: the endometriosis: Natural History, Diagnosis and Outcomes Study. Fertility and Sterility. 2013;**100**(1):162-9. e1-162-9.e2

[112] Itoh H, Iwasaki M, Hanaoka T, Sasaki H, Tanaka T, Tsugane S. Urinary bisphenol-A concentration in infertile Japanese women and its association with endometriosis: A cross-sectional study. Environmental Health and Preventive Medicine. 2007;**12**(6):258-264

[113] Simonelli A, Guadagni R, De Franciscis P, Colacurci N, Pieri M, Basilicata P, et al. Environmental and occupational exposure to bisphenol A and endometriosis: Urinary and peritoneal fluid concentration levels. International Archives of Occupational and Environmental Health. 2017;**90**(1):49-61

[114] Upson K, Sathyanarayana S, De Roos AJ, Koch HM, Scholes D, Holt VL. A population-based case-control study of urinary bisphenol A concentrations and risk of endometriosis. Human Reproduction (Oxford, England). 2014;**29**(11):2457-2464

[115] Rashidi BH, Amanlou M, Lak TB, Ghazizadeh M, Eslami B. A case-control study of bisphenol A and endometrioma among subgroup of Iranian women. Journal of Research in Medical Sciences: The Official Journal of Isfahan University of Medical Sciences. 2017;**22**:7

[116] Kendziorski JA, Belcher SM. Strain-specific induction of endometrial periglandular fibrosis in mice exposed during adulthood to the endocrine disrupting chemical bisphenol A. Reproductive Toxicology. 2015;**58**:119-130

[117] Signorile PG, Spugnini EP, Mita L, Mellone P, D'Avino A, Bianco M, et al. Pre-natal exposure of mice to bisphenol a elicits an endometriosis-like phenotype in female offspring. General and Comparative Endocrinology. 2010;**168**(3):318-325

[118] Reddy BS, Rozati R, Reddy S, Kodampur S, Reddy P, Reddy R. High plasma concentrations of polychlorinated biphenyls and phthalate esters in women with endometriosis: A prospective case control study. Fertility and Sterility. 2006;**85**(3):775-779

[119] Kim SH, Cho S, Ihm HJ, Oh YS, Heo SH, Chun S, et al. Possible role of phthalate in the pathogenesis of endometriosis: In vitro, animal, and

human data. The Journal of Clinical Endocrinology and Metabolism. 2015;**100**(12):E1502-E1511

[120] Weuve J, Hauser R, Calafat AM, Missmer SA, Wise LA. Association of exposure to phthalates with endometriosis and uterine leiomyomata: Findings from NHANES, 1999-2004. Environmental Health Perspectives. 2010;**118**(6):825-832

[121] Upson K, Sathyanarayana S, De Roos AJ, Thompson ML, Scholes D, Dills R, et al. Phthalates and risk of endometriosis. Environmental Research. 2013;**126**:91-97

[122] Moreira Fernandez MA, Cardeal ZL, Carneiro MM, André LC. Study of possible association between endometriosis and phthalate and bisphenol A by biomarkers analysis. Journal of Pharmaceutical and Biomedical Analysis. 2019;**172**:238-242

Section 2

Diagnosis of Endometriosis

Chapter 3

microRNA and Overcoming the Challenges of Their Use in the Diagnosis of Endometriosis

Victoria Turpin, Anna Leonova, Sanjay K. Agarwal and Warren G. Foster

Abstract

Endometriosis is a common estrogen dependent and inflammatory disease affecting approximately 176 million women worldwide. Currently, the time between onset of symptoms and a definitive diagnosis has been reported by several international studies to range from 6 to 12 years. Presently, laparoscopic surgery followed by histopathological confirmation of lesions remains the gold standard for diagnosis. In part because of cost and invasiveness, current trends favor reduced laparoscopic surgeries in preference of the non-surgical diagnosis of endometriosis. However, the search for a clinical marker or markers of endometriosis that provide equal or similar sensitivity and specificity to laparoscopy has remained elusive. Thus, the search for a diagnostic test for the diagnosis of endometriosis continues to be a high priority research and clinical issue. Recent studies have reported favorable results with microRNA; however, lack of replication and absence of validation suggest that circulating miRNA may not be reliable for clinical use. Use of different screening platforms together with divergent methods may account for some of the lack or reproducibility in the literature. Herein we critically assess the recent literature and explore sources for discrepant findings. We suggest that prospective studies using validated reference miRNA to normalize results together with improved study design may yet reveal a suitable diagnostic marker or panel of markers for the diagnosis of endometriosis.

Keywords: microRNA, miRNA, diagnosis, plasma, endometriosis

1. Background

Endometriosis is a common estrogen dependent and progesterone resistant disease of unknown cause characterized by growth of endometrial cells outside the uterine cavity [1]. It is estimated that 6–11% of all women are affected by endometriosis reaching an estimated 176 million women globally [2]. A chronic painful disease [3], endometriosis causes substantial health distress and interference with normal activities including work resulting in an average loss of 10.8 h/week from work [2] all leading to diminished quality of life (QOL) for affected women and their families. Chronic pelvic pain and infertility are common symptoms of endometriosis that bring women with this disease to seek medical attention. Approximately 71–87% of all women experiencing chronic pelvic pain and 50% of infertile women are diagnosed with endometriosis [4]. Thus, women with endometriosis report significant health distress and interference with normal activities including work and leisure time activities all leading to a deleterious effect upon women's social functioning, emotional well-being, employment, and vitality [5].

An important obstacle to the timely diagnosis and effective management of endometriosis is the lack of a simple diagnostic test. Diagnosis has been reported to be delayed by between 6 and 12 years with an average of 9 years from the onset of symptoms to definitive diagnosis [6]. Hence, identification of a clinical tool for the diagnosis of endometriosis has become a high priority research objective [2, 7, 8]. Health care providers and patients face a number of challenges in arriving at a diagnosis of endometriosis including: early age at onset of symptoms, normalization of pain by primary care providers, and suppression of symptoms through intermittent use of oral contraceptive pills [9]. Symptoms of endometriosis are shared with many other diseases including autoimmune diseases, cancer, irritable bowel syndrome (IBS), and musculoskeletal abnormalities. Therefore, an ideal biomarker of endometriosis must differentiate between endometriosis and other explanations for patient symptoms. In addition, clinical markers should be as minimally invasive as possible, affordable and convenient to use with the added benefit of providing insight into potential treatment response. Furthermore, the ideal biomarker must provide equivalent or similar outcome measures of sensitivity, specificity, positive, and negative predictive values to laparoscopy.

Currently, the gold standard for diagnosis remains visualization of endometriotic lesions typically by laparoscopy followed by histopathological confirmation of disease [10]. Current trends favoring the non-surgical diagnosis of endometriosis increase the pressure to identify novel clinical markers of endometriosis. Despite a plethora of biochemical differences in the peripheral circulation, peritoneal fluid, and endometrial tissues of women with endometriosis compared to healthy controls, no marker has been found with adequate sensitivity or specificity to challenge laparoscopy for the diagnosis of endometriosis whether used alone or in a panel of clinical markers [11–16]. However, reports of promising results have been brought forward in the literature from which epigenetic markers are potentially the most exciting.

2. Candidate clinical markers of endometriosis

Multiple gene and protein expression levels have been documented in women with endometriosis compared to controls; however, none have yielded reliable clinical markers of disease. Recent studies investigating the mechanisms controlling gene expression have produced promising results. Several histone modifications have been associated with endometriosis. For example, endometriotic stromal cells (ESC) have a lower global acetylation level of H3, and histone deacetylases 1 and 2 (HDAC1 and HDAC2) were upregulated compared to women without endometriosis [17]. Furthermore, histone deacetylase inhibitor (HDACI) treatment promoted apoptosis by reactivating the silenced chromatin [18]. G-protein-coupled estrogen receptor (GPER) expression and proliferation of endometriotic cells was inhibited by treatment with the HDACI's romidepsin and vorinostat [19]. These data suggest that histone modifications are involved in the pathophysiology of endometriosis and that HDACI's are promising agents for endometriosis treatment. However, use of histone markers in the diagnosis of endometriosis has yet to be explored.

Long-chain non-coding RNA (lnc-RNAs) are 200–100,000 bp RNA molecules which do not encode for protein, but are involved in transcriptional and post-transcriptional regulation of gene expression [20]. They are the most common non-coding RNAs and are involved in cell proliferation, differentiation, and apoptosis; all processes central in the pathobiology of endometriosis [21]. Some lnc-RNAs proposed as diagnostic markers of endometriosis include: H19 [22], CHL1-AS2

[23, 24], AC002454.1 [25], lncRNA SRA (steroid receptor RNA activator) [26], MALAT-1 [27], and LINC01279 [28]. Results of a recent study revealed the lnc-RNA are carried in circulating extracellular vesicles in women with endometriosis [29]. However, use of lnc-RNAs in the diagnosis of endometriosis has not been evaluated in a prospective study of women with symptoms suggestive of endometriosis with an independent validation step and thus their clinical utility remains uncertain.

Several recent studies have documented aberrant expression of multiple microRNAs (miRNAs) in the eutopic and ectopic endometrium of women with endometriosis [30–37]. miRNAs are short non-coding RNAs, 19–25 nucleotides long, that negatively regulate mRNA translation by repressing the protein translational machinery or degrading their target transcripts. Greater than 2000 mature human miRNA sequences have been identified and are thought to regulate approximately 50% of all protein coding genes. Multiple recent studies have documented differential microRNA (miRNA) expression in endometriotic tissues compared to eutopic endometrium of women with endometriosis and controls [33, 38–40]. miRNA are thought to hold promise as diagnostic biomarkers of disease because they are post-transcriptional regulators of gene expression that are stably expressed over time in bodily fluids and tissues [41]. Briefly, miRNA regulate protein expression through binding to and inhibiting the translation of mRNA transcripts into protein [42]. miRNAs are synthesized in the cytoplasm from nucleic hairpin intermediates (pre-miRNA) [43] which are then processed to yield mature miRNA that resist RNase degradation [41]. miRNA form an RNA-induced silencing complex (RISC) with Argonaute, Dicer, TAR RNA binding protein (TRBP) and protein activator of PKR (PACT) to post-transcriptionally regulate genes by binding to the 3′ region of the mRNA transcript and inhibiting translation [44].

In the early 2000s, several studies proposed that circulating levels of miRNA are differentially expressed in women with endometriosis compared to controls and thus could have diagnostic value [30, 31, 45]. Different methods including *in situ* hybridization, targeted RT-PCR and several different screening platforms including miRNA based microarrays, next generation sequencing and bio-informatics followed by RT-PCR validation have subsequently revealed a broad spectrum of miRNAs that are differentially expressed in women with endometriosis compared to control groups [29–31, 45–56]. However, to date, only the results for hsa-miR-451a [47, 48], 199a-5p [31, 54] and hsa-miR-141-3p [31, 49] have been successfully replicated in more than one study (**Table 1**). For the vast majority of miRNAs, differential expression has only been reported in a single study or the results for a few miRNAs have not been replicated by other investigators. For example, circulating levels of hsa-miR-145 were lower in women with endometriosis compared to controls [31] whereas hsa-miR-145 levels did not differ [47] or were higher in women with endometriosis compared to the control groups [50]. We postulate that divergent results may be the consequence of different screening platforms and technologies used to identify candidate miRNA markers of disease [57–59] and control group characteristics. Moreover, we suggest that different reference material used to quantify circulating miRNA levels are an additional source of variation.

While RNU6 has been widely used in the general miRNA literature to normalize miRNA expression in tissue, abundance and stability of expression have not been evaluated for circulating miRNA expression in women with endometriosis. Furthermore, RNU6 has low stability and abundance that is greatly influenced by sample storage and processing and the Cp values of RNU6 are highly variable from miRNA Cp values [51, 60, 61]. Similarly, the abundance and stability of miR-16-5p levels in the serum of women with endometriosis is uncertain but variable from the Cp values of miRNA targets [51]. Furthermore, circulating levels of miR-16-5p are altered by inflammation and stress [62, 63] and thus we suggest that both RNU6 and miR-16-5p are not suitable for normalization of circulating miRNA levels in women with endometriosis.

Fluid	Case/ control (N)	Cases	Controls	Reference miRNA	Cycle stage	Differentially expressed hsa-miR's	Citation
Serum	60/25	Stages I–IV	Symptomatic	RNU6	NS	↑**199a** and **122**, ↓9*, **145***, **141***, and 542-3p	[31]
Serum	24/24	Stage III and IV	Symptomatic	RNU6	P vs. S	↓let-7b, c, d, e, f (P) and 135a (S)	[46]
Serum	24/24	Stage III and IV	Symptomatic	RNU6	NS	↓3613-5p and 6755-3p ↑18a-5p, 125b-5p, 143-3p, 150-5p 342-3p, **451a** and 500a-3p	[47]
Serum	41/40	Stages I–IV	Symptomatic (n = 20) and Healthy (n = 20)	RNU6	NS	↑**451a**	[48]
Serum	30/20	Stages I–II	Infertile	cel-miR-39	ND	↓30c-5p, 127-3p, 99b-5p, 15b-5p, 20a-5p, and ↑424-3p, 185-5p	[52]
Serum	45/35	Stages I–IV	Symptomatic	RNU6	ND	↑**122** and **199a**	[54]
Serum	40/25	Stages I–IV	Healthy	18 s mRNA	ND	↓199a-5p	[55]
Plasma	23/23	Stage III and IV	Symptomatic	miR-16	ND	↓17-5p, 20a and 22	[30]
Plasma	61/30	Stages I–IV	Symptomatic (n = 35) and Healthy (n = 30)	miR-30e and 99a	NS	↓200a-3p and **141-3p**	[49]
Plasma	55/23	Stages I–IV	Symptomatic	miR-103-3p	ND	↑**145** (stages I and II), ↓31(stages I–IV)	[50]
Plasma	Variable	Stage I–IV	Symptomatic (n = 8–39) Healthy (n = 8)	RNU6 vs. miR-16 vs. miR-30b	NS	↓139-3p, 155 and 574-3p	[51]
Plasma	51/41	Stages I–IV	Symptomatic	miR-106a-5p, 199a-3p, 150-5p, 425-5p, 125a-5p, and 30e-5p	NS	↓miR154-5p and 378a-3p, ↑196b-5p and 33a-5p	[53]
Plasma	60/30	Stages I–IV	Symptomatic	miR-28-3p and 423-3p	S	*125b-5p, 28-5p, 29a-3p	[56]

Fluid	Case/ control (N)	Cases	Controls	Reference miRNA	Cycle stage	Differentially expressed hsa-miR's	Citation
Plasma	33/20	NR	Healthy	miR-132	NR	↑15b, 16, 191, 195, 1973, 1979, and 4284	[45]
Plasma	6/4	Stages III–IV	Healthy	RNU6	NR	↓375, 27a-3p, and 30d-5p	[29]

miRNA in bold have been replicated by at least one other group of investigators.
S = significant effect of menstrual cycle stage, NS = not significant, ND = not determined, NR = not reported, differential miR expression was either increased (↑) or decreased (↓) in women with endometriosis compared to controls.
**Direction could not be ascertained from the published report.*

Table 1.
Summary of miRNA's differentially expressed by microarray and RT-PCR in women with endometriosis (cases) compared to controls.

3. Effect of reference miRNA used to normalize results

While serum RNU6 has been widely used as the reference miRNA in prior endometriosis studies [29, 31, 46–48, 54], its levels have previously been reported to be unstable, unreliable, and a poor reference for miRNA since it is not processed or protected in the same way as miRNA [61, 63]. Therefore, we suggest that choice of reference miRNA can influence ability to detect significant differences and the direction of significant differences elicited. Previous studies report that hsa-miR-451a is upregulated in women with endometriosis compared to symptomatic controls [47] and compared to both symptomatic and asymptomatic (healthy) control groups [48]. Both prior studies employed RNU6 as a reference. While hsa-miR-451a has been found to act as a tumor suppressor [64, 65], it is also a marker of hemolysis [66] and thus we suggest that care should be employed to exclude samples with hemolysis before analysis. The miRNA ratio of hsa-miR-451a and hsa-miR-23a-3p has been employed by others [56, 67] to monitor for sample hemolysis. Therefore, we suggest that hsa-miR-451a has limited value as a candidate marker of endometriosis.

4. Effect of control group definition

Several studies have employed healthy women as their control population [29, 45, 48, 49, 51, 55], thus allowing circulating miRNA levels in women with endometriosis to be compared to symptomatic and asymptomatic healthy control populations. While the majority of previous reports employed symptomatic controls [30, 31, 46–51, 53, 54, 56], hsa-miR-16-5p [30, 51] RNU6 (the most common) reference material used to normalize miRNA expression [31, 46–48, 51, 54]; reference materials that are unsuitable for normalizing serum miRNA expression. In our experience, differential miRNA expression was dependent upon whether comparisons were made with asymptomatic compared to symptomatic controls. Therefore, we suggest that control group characteristics on the differential expression of candidate miRNA in women with endometriosis merits further investigation.

While, lack of replication, absence of validation of results, and poor sensitivity and specificity currently limit the value of miRNA as diagnostic markers of endometriosis [51], we propose that usefulness of miRNA for the diagnosis of endometriosis cannot be evaluated without appropriate determination of appropriate reference miRNA.

5. Future directions

Although identification of clinical markers of endometriosis has long been sought, none has so far been suitable to displace laparoscopy as the gold standard for diagnosis. Endometriosis is a complex heterogenous disease with variable presentation whose symptoms are easily confused with other clinical problems. Since endometriosis is detectable with high frequency amongst asymptomatic women [68] surgical exclusion of disease in the control group is essential to prevent biasing results towards the null. Consequently, we suggest that control or reference group definition is important. Numerous prior studies reporting differential miRNA expression in women with endometriosis have employed asymptomatic women as their reference population [29, 45, 48, 49, 51, 55]. However, healthy women without symptoms of endometriosis and without evidence of endometriosis by laparoscopy (asymptomatic control) and symptomatic women without evidence of disease at the time of laparoscopy (symptomatic control) are functionally different, yet both groups continue to be employed as controls in contemporary studies. Results from our laboratory suggest that inclusion of asymptomatic controls can produce misleading results and thus speculate that restricting the control group to symptomatic controls in future studies may improve reproducibility of results. In addition to control group, we propose that the use of validated reference miRNA to normalize results also affects detection of levels of miRNA differentially expressed in women with endometriosis compared to controls.

Having identified candidate miRNA for the diagnosis of endometriosis it will be important to determine their relationship with pelvic pain as well as response to treatment. In the absence of this data the potential prognostic value of candidate markers of endometriosis remains uncertain. We also propose that future studies with robust sample size will be needed to clarify the relationship between circulating miRNA levels and menstrual cycle phase. Studies reporting menstrual cycle stage and circulating miRNA levels are thus far have produced equivocal results [31, 46–49, 51, 53, 56]. Furthermore, lesion type (endometrioma, peritoneal endometriosis, deep infiltrating endometriosis) are biologically distinct and thus a single clinical marker is unlikely to be dysregulated in all lesion types and thus a panel of markers may be more relevant. Furthermore, duration of disease and age of lesion may also present with functional differences. Therefore, discovery of clinical markers should describe the lesion types present in study participants. The influence of study participant age and body mass index are also important variables associated with pelvic pain and disease severity that are frequently not considered in analyses of clinical markers of endometriosis. Finally, the functional role of candidate markers in endometriosis has the potential to suggest therapeutic targets for additional research.

6. Summary and conclusions

Use of reference miRNA that may not be ideal for normalization of results may account for noted weaknesses in the literature. Use of validated reference miRNA markers and careful control of sample condition for potential confounders should improve study replication. Finally, although circulating miRNA levels have low variability in women with endometriosis, it will be necessary for discovery phases to include a large number of study participants to control for participant age, menstrual cycle stage, BMI, stage of disease, and type of lesions. Thus, we suggest that despite set-backs with reproducibility of results, it may be too soon to judge the diagnostic potential of miRNA.

Acknowledgements

Funding support for this project was provided by a research operating grant (MOP142230) from the Canadian Institutes of Health Research to WGF. The authors are grateful to Ms. Annette Bullen for her assistance in study participant recruitment, access to clinical data, and sample collection. The assistance of the Endo@Mac surgical team (Drs. Nick Leyland, Sarah Scatollon, and Dustin Costescu) with access to study participants, staging of disease, and collection of blood samples is greatly appreciated.

Author details

Victoria Turpin[1], Anna Leonova[1], Sanjay K. Agarwal[2] and Warren G. Foster[1,2]*

1 Department of Obstetrics and Gynecology, McMaster University, Hamilton, Ontario, Canada

2 Department of Obstetrics, Gynecology and Reproductive Sciences, University of California, San Diego, California, United States of America

*Address all correspondence to: fosterw@mcmaster.ca

References

[1] Sampson J. Peritoneal endometriosis due to the menstrual dissemination of endometrial tissue into the peritoneal cavity. American Journal of Obstetrics and Gynecology. 1927;**14**:422-469

[2] Rogers PA, Adamson GD, Al-Jefout M, Becker CM, D'Hooghe TM, Dunselman GA, et al. Research priorities for endometriosis. Reproductive Sciences. 2017;**24**(2):202-226

[3] Kennedy S, Bergqvist A, Chapron C, D'Hooghe T, Dunselman G, Greb R, et al. ESHRE guideline for the diagnosis and treatment of endometriosis. Human Reproduction. 2005;**20**(10):2698-2704

[4] Aredo JV, Heyrana KJ, Karp BI, Shah JP, Stratton P. Relating chronic pelvic pain and endometriosis to signs of sensitization and myofascial pain and dysfunction. Seminars in Reproductive Medicine. 2017;**35**(1):88-97

[5] Jones G, Jenkinson C, Kennedy S. The impact of endometriosis upon quality of life: A qualitative analysis. Journal of Psychosomatic Obstetrics & Gynecology. 2004;**25**(2):123-133

[6] Agarwal SK, Chapron C, Giudice LC, Laufer MR, Leyland N, Missmer SA, et al. Clinical diagnosis of endometriosis: A call to action. American Journal of Obstetrics and Gynecology. 2019;**220**(4):354.e351-354.e312

[7] Rogers PA, D'Hooghe TM, Fazleabas A, Giudice LC, Montgomery GW, Petraglia F, et al. Defining future directions for endometriosis research: Workshop report from the 2011 world congress of endometriosis in Montpellier, France. Reproductive Sciences. 2013;**20**(5):483-499

[8] Rogers PA, D'Hooghe TM, Fazleabas A, Gargett CE, Giudice LC, Montgomery GW, et al. Priorities for endometriosis research: Recommendations from an international consensus workshop. Reproductive Sciences. 2009;**16**(4):335-346

[9] Ballard K, Lowton K, Wright J. What's the delay? A qualitative study of women's experiences of reaching a diagnosis of endometriosis. Fertility and Sterility. 2006;**86**(5):1296-1301

[10] Wykes CB, Clark TJ, Khan KS. Accuracy of laparoscopy in the diagnosis of endometriosis: A systematic quantitative review. BJOG. 2004;**111**(11):1204-1212

[11] May KE, Conduit-Hulbert SA, Villar J, Kirtley S, Kennedy SH, Becker CM. Peripheral biomarkers of endometriosis: A systematic review. Human Reproduction Update. 2010;**16**(6):651-674

[12] May KE, Villar J, Kirtley S, Kennedy SH, Becker CM. Endometrial alterations in endometriosis: A systematic review of putative biomarkers. Human Reproduction Update. 2011;**17**(5):637-653

[13] Fassbender A, Burney RO, O DF, D'Hooghe T, Giudice L. Update on biomarkers for the detection of endometriosis. BioMed Research International. 2015;**2015**:130854

[14] Fassbender A, Vodolazkaia A, Saunders P, Lebovic D, Waelkens E, De MB, et al. Biomarkers of endometriosis. Fertility and Sterility. 2013;**99**(4):1135-1145

[15] Toor K, Wessels JM, Agarwal SK, Leyland N, Foster WG. Clinical markers of endometriosis: Have we been too quick to judge? Medical Hypotheses. 2014;**82**(4):493-501

[16] Nisenblat V, Bossuyt PM, Shaikh R, Farquhar C, Jordan V, Scheffers CS,

et al. Blood biomarkers for the non-invasive diagnosis of endometriosis. Cochrane Database of Systematic Reviews. 2016;**5**:CD012179

[17] Monteiro JB, Colón-Díaz M, García M, Gutierrez S, Colón M, Seto E, et al. Endometriosis is characterized by a distinct pattern of histone 3 and histone 4 lysine modifications. Reproductive Sciences. 2014;**21**(3):305-318

[18] Cameron EE, Bachman KE, Myöhänen S, Herman JG, Baylin SB. Synergy of demethylation and histone deacetylase inhibition in the re-expression of genes silenced in cancer. Nature Genetics. 1999;**21**(1):103-107

[19] Imesch P, Samartzis EP, Dedes KJ, Fink D, Fedier A. Histone deacetylase inhibitors down-regulate G-protein-coupled estrogen receptor and the GPER-antagonist G-15 inhibits proliferation in endometriotic cells. Fertility and Sterility. 2013;**100**(3):770-776

[20] Spizzo R, Almeida MI, Colombatti A, Calin GA. Long non-coding RNAs and cancer: A new frontier of translational research? Oncogene. 2012;**31**(43):4577-4587

[21] Johnsson P, Lipovich L, Grandér D, Morris KV. Evolutionary conservation of long non-coding RNAs; sequence, structure, function. Biochimica et Biophysica Acta. 2014;**1840**(3):1063-1071

[22] Ghazal S, McKinnon B, Zhou J, Mueller M, Men Y, Yang L, et al. H19 lncRNA alters stromal cell growth via IGF signaling in the endometrium of women with endometriosis. EMBO Molecular Medicine. 2015;7(8):996-1003

[23] Sun PR, Jia SZ, Lin H, Leng JH, Lang JH. Genome-wide profiling of long noncoding ribonucleic acid expression patterns in ovarian endometriosis by microarray. Fertility and Sterility. 2014;**101**(4):1038-1046.e1037

[24] Zhang C, Wu W, Ye X, Ma R, Luo J, Zhu H, et al. Aberrant expression of CHL1 gene and long non-coding RNA CHL1-AS1, CHL1-AS2 in ovarian endometriosis. European Journal of Obstetrics, Gynecology, and Reproductive Biology. 2019;**236**:177-182

[25] Wang Y, Li Y, Yang Z, Liu K, Wang D. Genome-wide microarray analysis of long non-coding RNAs in Eutopic secretory endometrium with endometriosis. Cellular Physiology and Biochemistry. 2015;**37**(6):2231-2245

[26] Lin K, Zhan H, Ma J, Xu K, Wu R, Zhou C, et al. Silencing of SRA1 regulates ER expression and attenuates the growth of stromal cells in ovarian endometriosis. Reproductive Sciences. 2017;**24**(6):836-843

[27] Liu H, Zhang Z, Xiong W, Zhang L, Du Y, Liu Y, et al. Long non-coding RNA MALAT1 mediates hypoxia-induced pro-survival autophagy of endometrial stromal cells in endometriosis. Journal of Cellular and Molecular Medicine. 2019;**23**(1):439-452

[28] Liu J, Wang Q, Zhang R, Zhang C, Lin J, Huang X. Identification of LINC01279 as a cell cycle-associated long non-coding RNA in endometriosis with GBA analysis. Molecular Medicine Reports. 2018;**18**(4):3850-3858

[29] Khalaj K, Miller JE, Lingegowda H, Fazleabas AT, Young SL, Lessey BA, et al. Extracellular vesicles from endometriosis patients are characterized by a unique miRNA-lncRNA signature. JCI Insight. 2019;**4**(18):e12886

[30] Jia SZ, Yang Y, Lang J, Sun P, Leng J. Plasma miR-17-5p, miR-20a and miR-22 are down-regulated in women with endometriosis. Human Reproduction. 2013;**28**(2):322-330

[31] Wang WT, Zhao YN, Han BW, Hong SJ, Chen YQ. Circulating microRNAs identified in a genome-wide serum microRNA expression analysis as noninvasive biomarkers for endometriosis. Journal of Clinical Endocrinology and Metabolism. 2013;**98**(1):281-289

[32] Liu S, Gao S, Wang XY, Wang DB. Expression of miR-126 and Crk in endometriosis: miR-126 may affect the progression of endometriosis by regulating Crk expression. Archives of Gynecology and Obstetrics. 2012;**285**(4):1065-1072

[33] Shen L, Yang S, Huang W, Xu W, Wang Q, Song Y, et al. MicroRNA23a and microRNA23b deregulation derepresses SF-1 and upregulates estrogen signaling in ovarian endometriosis. Journal of Clinical Endocrinology and Metabolism. 2013;**98**(4):1575-1582

[34] Ramon LA, Braza-Boils A, Gilabert-Estelles J, Gilabert J, Espana F, Chirivella M, et al. microRNAs expression in endometriosis and their relation to angiogenic factors. Human Reproduction. 2011;**26**(5):1082-1090

[35] Gilabert-Estelles J, Braza-Boils A, Ramon LA, Zorio E, Medina P, Espana F, et al. Role of microRNAs in gynecological pathology. Current Medicinal Chemistry. 2012;**19**(15):2406-2413

[36] Braza-Boils A, Mari-Alexandre J, Gilabert J, Sanchez-Izquierdo D, Espana F, Estelles A, et al. MicroRNA expression profile in endometriosis: Its relation to angiogenesis and fibrinolytic factors. Human Reproduction. 2014;**29**(5):978-988

[37] Braza-Boils A, Gilabert-Estelles J, Ramon LA, Gilabert J, Mari-Alexandre J, Chirivella M, et al. Peritoneal fluid reduces angiogenesis-related microRNA expression in cell cultures of endometrial and endometriotic tissues from women with endometriosis. PLoS ONE. 2013;**8**(4):e62370

[38] Haikalis ME, Wessels JM, Leyland NA, Agarwal SK, Foster WG. miRNA expression pattern differs depending on endometriosis lesion type. Biology of Reproduction. 2018;**98**(5):623-633

[39] Burney RO, Hamilton AE, Aghajanova L, Vo KC, Nezhat CN, Lessey BA, et al. MicroRNA expression profiling of eutopic secretory endometrium in women with versus without endometriosis. Molecular Human Reproduction. 2009;**15**(10):625-631

[40] Laudanski P, Charkiewicz R, Tolwinska A, Szamatowicz J, Charkiewicz A, Niklinski J. Profiling of selected MicroRNAs in proliferative Eutopic endometrium of women with ovarian endometriosis. BioMed Research International. 2015;**2015**:760698

[41] Chen X, Ba Y, Ma L, Cai X, Yin Y, Wang K, et al. Characterization of microRNAs in serum: A novel class of biomarkers for diagnosis of cancer and other diseases. Cell Research. 2008;**18**(10):997-1006

[42] Bartel DP. MicroRNAs: Genomics, biogenesis, mechanism, and function. Cell. 2004;**116**(2):281-297

[43] Lee Y, Jeon K, Lee JT, Kim S, Kim VN. MicroRNA maturation: Stepwise processing and subcellular localization. The EMBO Journal. 2002;**21**(17):4663-4670

[44] Chendrimada TP, Gregory RI, Kumaraswamy E, Norman J, Cooch N, Nishikura K, et al. TRBP recruits the dicer complex to Ago2 for microRNA processing and gene silencing. Nature. 2005;**436**(7051):740-744

[45] Suryawanshi S, Vlad AM, Lin HM, Mantia-Smaldone G, Laskey R, Lee M,

et al. Plasma microRNAs as novel biomarkers for endometriosis and endometriosis-associated ovarian cancer. Clinical Cancer Research. 2013;**19**(5):1213-1224

[46] Cho S, Mutlu L, Grechukhina O, Taylor HS. Circulating microRNAs as potential biomarkers for endometriosis. Fertility and Sterility. 2015;**103**(5):1252-1260 e1251

[47] Cosar E, Mamillapalli R, Ersoy GS, Cho S, Seifer B, Taylor HS. Serum microRNAs as diagnostic markers of endometriosis: A comprehensive array-based analysis. Fertility and Sterility. 2016;**106**(2):402-409

[48] Nothnick WB, Falcone T, Joshi N, Fazleabas AT, Graham A. Serum miR-451a levels are significantly elevated in women with endometriosis and recapitulated in baboons (*Papio anubis*) with experimentally-induced disease. Reproductive Sciences. 2017;**24**(8):1195-1202

[49] Rekker K, Saare M, Roost AM, Kaart T, Soritsa D, Karro H, et al. Circulating miR-200-family micro-RNAs have altered plasma levels in patients with endometriosis and vary with blood collection time. Fertility and Sterility. 2015;**104**(4):938-946 e932

[50] Bashti O, Noruzinia M, Garshasbi M, Abtahi M. miR-31 and miR-145 as potential non-invasive regulatory biomarkers in patients with endometriosis. Cell Journal. 2018;**20**(2):293

[51] Nisenblat V, Sharkey DJ, Wang Z, Evans SF, Healey M, Ohlsson Teague EMC, et al. Plasma microRNAs display limited potential as diagnostic tools for endometriosis. The Journal of Clinical Endocrinology and Metabolism. 2019;**104**(6):1999-2022

[52] Wang L, Huang W, Ren C, Zhao M, Jiang X, Fang X, et al. Analysis of serum microRNA profile by Solexa sequencing in women with endometriosis. Reproductive Sciences. 2016;**23**(10):1359-1370

[53] Pateisky P, Pils D, Szabo L, Kuessel L, Husslein H, Schmitz A, et al. Hsa-miRNA-154-5p expression in plasma of endometriosis patients is a potential diagnostic marker for the disease. Reproductive Biomedicine Online. 2018;**37**(4):449-466

[54] Maged AM, Deeb WS, El Amir A, Zaki SS, El Sawah H, Al Mohamady M, et al. Diagnostic accuracy of serum miR-122 and miR-199a in women with endometriosis. International Journal of Gynaecology and Obstetrics. 2018;**141**(1):14-19

[55] Hsu CY, Hsieh TH, Tsai CF, Tsai HP, Chen HS, Chang Y, et al. miRNA-199a-5p regulates VEGFA in endometrial mesenchymal stem cells and contributes to the pathogenesis of endometriosis. The Journal of Pathology. 2014;**232**(3):330-343

[56] Vanhie A, O D, Peterse D, Beckers A, Cuéllar A, Fassbender A, et al. Plasma miRNAs as biomarkers for endometriosis. Human Reproduction. 2019;**34**(9):1650-1660

[57] Mestdagh P, Hartmann N, Baeriswyl L, Andreasen D, Bernard N, Chen C, et al. Evaluation of quantitative miRNA expression platforms in the microRNA quality control (miRQC) study. Nature Methods. 2014;**11**(8):809-815

[58] Kok MGM, de Ronde MWJ, Moerland PD, Ruijter JM, Creemers EE, Pinto-Sietsma SJ. Small sample sizes in high-throughput miRNA screens: A common pitfall for the identification of miRNA biomarkers. Biomolecular Detection and Quantification. 2018;**15**:1-5

[59] Pritchard CC, Cheng HH, Tewari M. MicroRNA profiling:

Approaches and considerations. Nature Reviews. Genetics. 2012;**13**(5):358-369

[60] Graham A, Falcone T, Nothnick WB. The expression of microRNA-451 in human endometriotic lesions is inversely related to that of macrophage migration inhibitory factor (MIF) and regulates MIF expression and modulation of epithelial cell survival. Human Reproduction. 2015;**30**(3):642-652

[61] Xiang M, Zeng Y, Yang R, Xu H, Chen Z, Zhong J, et al. U6 is not a suitable endogenous control for the quantification of circulating microRNAs. Biochemical and Biophysical Research Communications. 2014;**454**(1):210-214

[62] Wang H, Zhang P, Chen W, Feng D, Jia Y, Xie LX. Evidence for serum miR-15a and miR-16 levels as biomarkers that distinguish sepsis from systemic inflammatory response syndrome in human subjects. Clinical Chemistry and Laboratory Medicine. 2012;**50**(8):1423-1428

[63] Katsuura S, Kuwano Y, Yamagishi N, Kurokawa K, Kajita K, Akaike Y, et al. MicroRNAs miR-144/144* and miR-16 in peripheral blood are potential biomarkers for naturalistic stress in healthy Japanese medical students. Neuroscience Letters. 2012;**516**(1):79-84

[64] Liu G, Xu Z, Hao D. MicroRNA-451 inhibits neuroblastoma proliferation, invasion and migration by targeting macrophage migration inhibitory factor. Molecular Medicine Reports. 2016;**13**(3):2253-2260

[65] Xu H, Mei Q, Shi L, Lu J, Zhao J, Fu Q. Tumor-suppressing effects of miR451 in human osteosarcoma. Cell Biochemistry and Biophysics. 2014;**69**(1):163-168

[66] Shkurnikov MY, Knyazev EN, Fomicheva KA, Mikhailenko DS, Nyushko KM, Saribekyan EK, et al. Analysis of plasma microRNA associated with Hemolysis. Bulletin of Experimental Biology and Medicine. 2016;**160**(6):748-750

[67] Blondal T, Jensby Nielsen S, Baker A, Andreasen D, Mouritzen P, Wrang Teilum M, et al. Assessing sample and miRNA profile quality in serum and plasma or other biofluids. Methods. 2013;**59**(1):S1-S6

[68] Rawson JM. Prevalence of endometriosis in asymptomatic women. Journal of Reproductive Medicine. 1991;**36**(7):513-515

Chapter 4

Pain Testing in Endometriosis for the Clinician

John Jarrell

Abstract

Clinical pain testing has been used to ascertain the pathophysiology of many clinical conditions, but its use in the management of endometriosis has been limited. Although the testing can require the use of complex testing in the laboratory, this chapter is directed to look at a test for allodynia that can be applied in the clinic. The test for cutaneous allodynia is validated, does not require sophisticated tools, and is readily accepted by woman. The presence of allodynia in certain gynecological presentations can indicate the woman's pain system has become sensitized. Uses of the test in clinical encounters with women suffering from endometriosis and possible uses in future are presented.

Keywords: pelvic pain, pain testing, pain sensitization, visceral pain, endometriosis

1. Introduction

The object of this chapter is to introduce and describe pain testing for gynecologists to use at the bedside. Although the subject's description of pain is still the best method of assessing pain, the use of objective pain measures permit independent quantification that is useful in explaining a more complete picture of a disease process, and it is also of help in documenting change in response to medical or surgical intervention. Formal pain testing has now provided new information on the pain mechanisms in chronic pancreatitis, dysmenorrhea, painful bladder syndrome, osteoporosis, and low back pain to name a few conditions [1–5]. Central sensitization has been identified as a component of persistent pelvic pain, with and without endometriosis [3–5]. This summary is intended to provide several examples where testing gives both the woman and the gynecologist a fuller appreciation of the clinical problem of pain.

Clinical pain testing has been used to ascertain the pathophysiology of many clinical conditions, but its use in the management of endometriosis has been limited. Although the testing can require the use of complex testing in the laboratory, this chapter is directed to look at a test for allodynia that can be applied in the clinic. The test for cutaneous allodynia is validated, does not require sophisticated tools, and is readily accepted by woman. The presence of allodynia in certain gynecological presentations can indicate the woman's pain system has become sensitized. Uses of the test in clinical encounters with women suffering from endometriosis and possible uses in future are presented.

2. Visceral pain physiology

The physiological basis for pain testing is viscero-somatic pain referral. One of the first such observations was made by Sir James Mackenzie (1853–1925). Although known primarily for his work on cardiac physiology, arrhythmias, and heart disease, he wrote a book in 1913 that provides insight into how we might understand the clinical signs of pelvic disease [6]. Mackenzie provided a diagram of a man with biliary colic who had pain radiating to his right upper quadrant (**Figure 1**). This painful area was also found to have an area of allodynia in the same area. Allodynia is defined as pain from a non-painful source. The allodynia can be static or dynamic depending on the mode of testing. Static allodynia is direct pressure on the skin, while dynamic allodynia uses movement across the affected area. Notably, Mackenzie found a small area within the region of allodynia that was particularly tender and corresponded to the anterior cutaneous nerve that passed through the abdominal wall fascia. Mackenzie correctly noted that not only the colicky pain was referred to the right upper quadrant but also there was also a tiny muscular component of this referral, centered on the tender ninth thoracic nerve as it perforates the abdominal wall fascia.

This simple diagram is the basis for the clinical testing of women's pelvic pain at the bedside. Most of the causes of pain in the pelvis associated with endometriosis are due to inflammatory processes. These are considered nociceptive influences on the afferent nervous system that pass to the spinal cord primarily in the T12 and L1 segments. The viscero-somatic referral then initiates efferent activity through the corresponding anterior cutaneous nerves to the lower abdomen. The result of the efferent activity is the pattern of allodynia and tender areas in a similar fashion to Mackenzie (**Figure 1**). There are many variations of the presentation, unilateral, bilateral, with both equal and unequal sizes of the allodynia [6].

Another contributor was Sir Henry Head (1861–1940) who, mapped out the referral patterns of the body of many illnesses that initially became the Head zones but later evolved to be the dermatomes. The accompanying figure demonstrates the ovarian zones (**Figure 2**) [7].

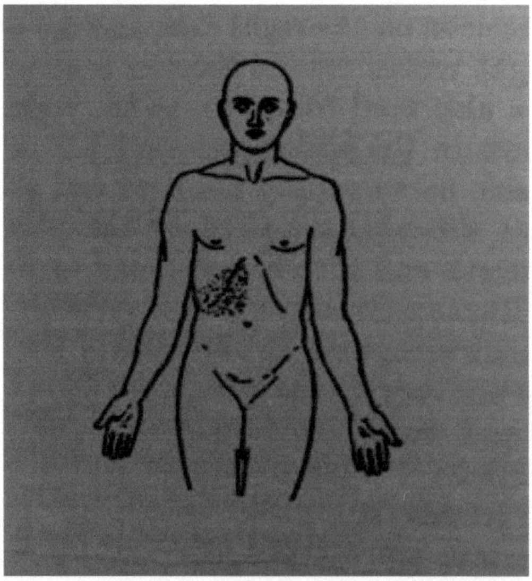

Figure 1.
Location of right upper quadrant allodynia associated with tenderness in the region of ninth anterior cutaneous nerve due to biliary colic.

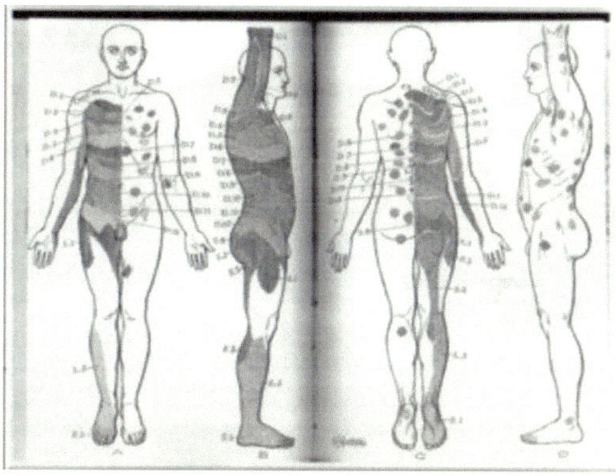

Figure 2.
Demonstration of the Head zones.

More recent studies of the visceral-somatic referral and guidelines for the management of associated persistent pain have been reported [8–12].

3. Detection of allodynia and expansion

To detect allodynia, a cotton-tipped applicator is slowly drawn down from the midclavicular line toward the pubic region along the imagined border of the rectus abdominus muscle. It is necessary to start the test outside the area of allodynia. Starting within will not detect the necessary changes. As the applicator is positioned, the woman is asked to note if there is any sudden change in sensation or the onset of a sharp pain. When this is announced, the level is marked off with a body marker. An example of two small areas of allodynia containing trigger points associated with the T12 anterior cutaneous nerves is shown in **Figure 3**.

An extreme example of severe chronic pelvic pain demonstrates how large the area of allodynia can become—this degree is unusual (**Figure 4**). The delineation of allodynia that is marked off with a pen can stimulate spinal activity such that there is an almost immediate shift in the borders of allodynia (**Figure 4**). These shifts in the levels of sensation correspond to "jumps" taking place in the spinal cord, segment by segment.

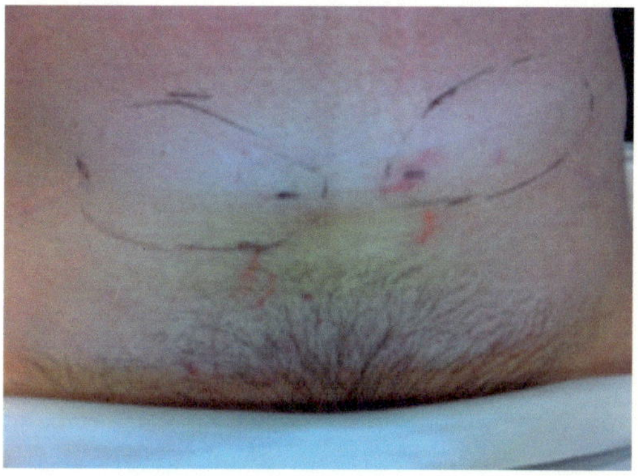

Figure 3.
Small areas of allodynia containing painful trigger points of T12 anterior cutaneous nerves.

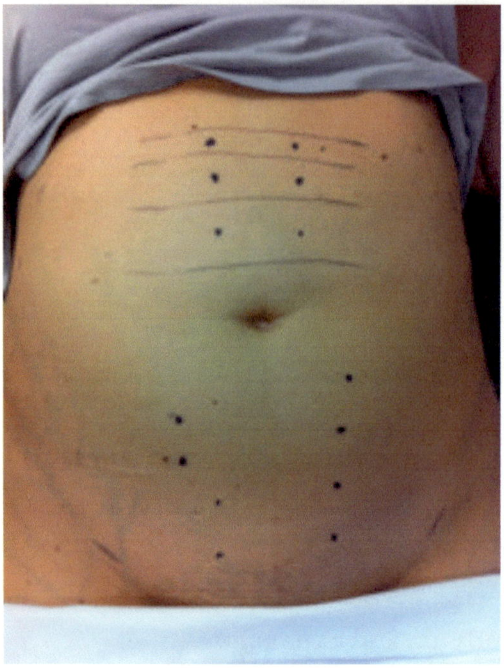

Figure 4.
An example of allodynia expansion upward by dermatome with each test for allodynia in a woman with severe pelvic pain.

4. Hyperalgesia and location of trigger points on the abdomen

Associated with the allodynia, one can determine the presence of hyperalgesia, which is an increased pain sensation from a painful source. The examining finger can detect this when gently applied to the area (**Figure 5**). The examination has to be gentle as a pressure of only 15–20 g can evoke severe pain from the small nodular trigger point (**Figure 5**). The location of the trigger point has been marked in **Figure 6**.

A more sophisticated way of determining the degree of hyperalgesia is with an algometer. This instrument will determine the pressure pain threshold. Measures of pressure pain thresholds are reduced in the areas affected by pain sensitization. In many cases of severe chronic pelvic pain, it is possible to put only the mildest

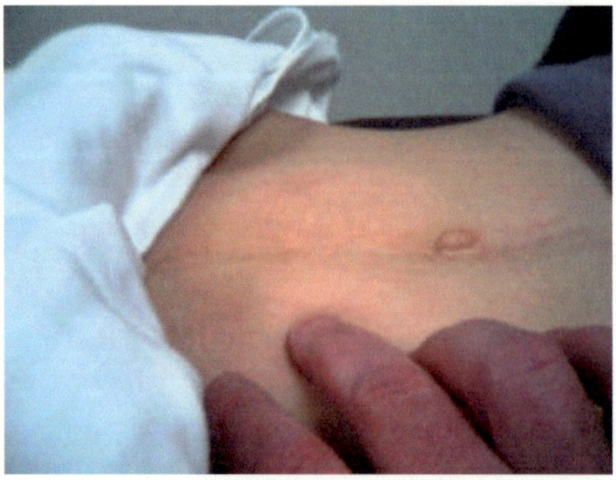

Figure 5.
Localizing a viscerally related trigger point with gentle pressure from the pulp of the examining finger.

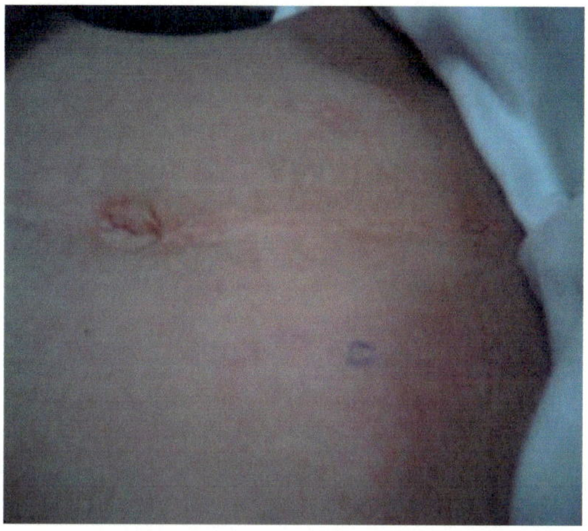

Figure 6.
The location of the trigger point corresponds to the right anterior cutaneous nerve from T12 spinal nerve.

pressure in the region of the anterior cutaneous nerve to have the induced pain threshold recorded.

5. Validity of allodynia testing in pelvic pain

In order to have faith in allodynia, it is important to ensure the test has reliability. In a cohort of 81 women with chronic pelvic pain, the presence of allodynia was significantly associated with those who were suffering from visceral disease [13].

The positive predictive values for pelvic visceral disease were as follows:

Abdominal cutaneous allodynia	93%
Perineal cutaneous allodynia	91%
Abdominal myofascial trigger points	93%
Perineal myofascial trigger points	81%
Reduced pain thresholds	79%

The likelihood ratio (+) and 95% C.I. for the detection of visceral sources of pain were as follows:

Abdominal cutaneous allodynia	4.19 (1.46, 12.0)
Perineal cutaneous allodynia	2.91 (1.19, 7.11)
Abdominal myofascial trigger points	4.19 (1.46, 12.0)
Pelvic myofascial trigger points	1.35 (0.86, 2.13)
Reduced pain thresholds	1.14 (0.85, 1.52), [13]

In another study of validity, a total of 22 females with chronic pelvic pain were compared to 23 pain-free controls and 12 cyclic pain patients. Participants were evaluated by two clinicians. Investigators mapped the abdomen with the cotton-tipped applicator, outlined the areas of allodynia with a body pen, photographed the abdomen, and wiped off the marking before the second investigator repeated the test. The interrater reliability resulted in 98% agreement for the three study groups. The cotton-tipped applicator test showed 73% sensitivity and 100% specificity for differentiating patients with chronic pelvic pain from pain-free patients [14]. At present, there do not appear to be pain-testing techniques that specifically identify endometriosis independent from other visceral diseases. It is arguable, however, that the experience of pain may have greater relevance depending on the clinical situation as described in relation to the negative laparoscopy.

6. The negative laparoscopy

A comparison of the results of pain testing was done in women investigated for pelvic pain between 69 with confirmed endometriosis compared to 35 who had a negative laparoscopy [15]. When women with a negative laparoscopy were compared to those with confirmed endometriosis, there were no differences in age, gravidity, parity, menarche, and frequency of dyspareunia or duration of severe dysmenorrhea. There were no differences in the frequency of abdominal wall allodynia or of pressure pain thresholds. These tests give validation to the women who otherwise have no explanation and it also raises the possibility that dysmenorrhea may be the source of the pelvic pain. These results are consistent with testing of women with persistent pelvic pain with and without endometriosis [3].

7. Prediction of postoperative pain

There has been a great deal of interest in the prediction of postoperative pain, but most of the studies have not included laparoscopic pelvic surgery. The situation is very complex with a wide number of variables having a role such as preoperative pain, depression, previous surgery, gender, and opiate use and abuse. A study of the assessment of predicting postoperative pain considered these elements but also included testing for the presence of allodynia and hyperalgesia before and after 6 months following laparoscopic surgery for non-acute pain. Hyperalgesia was identified with the use of a Somedic Algometer (Somedic SenseLab AB, Norra Mellby 1129 SE-280 10 Sösdala, Sweden). In women who underwent tubal ligation, pain levels were low before and after the procedure. In 61 women who underwent surgery for non-acute pain, pain levels at 6 months and all psychologic test scores were reduced significantly compared with baseline ($P < .001$ and $P = .001$, respectively). Among those women with positive results on the quantitative pain tests of sensitization at baseline, average postoperative pain was also significantly reduced ($P < .001$). Univariate analysis demonstrated only tests of sensitization were correlated with the reduction in average pain level ($P = .01$). Regression analysis suggested that baseline pain, catastrophizing, and the presence of cutaneous allodynia significantly predicted pain levels after 6 months. We had anticipated sensitization would have predicted more pain, but we have interpreted the results to indicate the reduction in pain may be due to the successful removal of a nociceptive source in the pelvis. At present, pain testing does not indicate whether surgery should or should not be done; that remains a clinical decision.

8. Detection of sensitization in relation to psychological status

Also, a secondary analysis reviewed the changes in pain and psychological measures of stress (Pain Disability Index, Pain Catastrophizing Scale, CES-D (Center for Epidemiologic Studies Depression Scale)), depression scale, and the McGill Pain Scale (short form) as the presence of pain sensitization. Preoperatively, the psychological test scores correlated significantly with the pain scores. Post-laparoscopic surgery pain and psychosocial test scores were reduced and remained significantly correlated. The presence of preoperative pain sensitization was associated with trends to greater baseline and 6-month postoperative changes in average pain and measures of psychological distress [16].

9. Relationship to pelvic floor

In a study of 112 women with chronic pelvic pain assessed for pain in the abdominal wall, perineum, levator ani, and obturator internus, the number of myofascial trigger points was predicted by the number of previous laparoscopies adjusted for age. Both the presence of visceral disease and endometriosis were significantly associated with higher numbers of myofascial dysfunction than the absence of these conditions [17]. These findings suggested that prior surgery may aggravate pain sensitization. The available studies using pain testing do not indicate they can discriminate endometriosis from other visceral diseases [3, 13, 18]. It should also be noted here the test for allodynia on the perineum was validated as noted above [13].

10. Possible future benefits of pain testing

It has long been known that the extent of disease does not have a correlation with the severity of pain. Many women with minimal disease are severely incapacitated with their pain. Alternatively, but less common, are women with severe stage 4 disease without pelvic pain. Many gynecologists have seen women who have had repeated procedures for minimal disease despite having no change in their pain [18]. The techniques of pain testing can provide an assessment indicating peripheral and central sensitization have altered pain physiology and possibly eliminate the need for repetitive laparoscopic surgery of limited, if any, benefit.

There have been several blinded controlled trials of the excision versus sham excision of endometriosis for the management of pain [19–22]. The results have differed; in several, there was a reduction in pain; in another that was extended out 14 years post-randomization, there was no difference between the sham excision and excision. Perhaps it may not be the surgeons' expertise, the degree of disease, or prior pelvic surgery, but the differences may possibly be explained by the womens' pain sensitization. Pain testing might have a unifying feature to allow comparisons of cohorts of subjects in clinical trials.

Many surgeons have had the unsettling experience of having one of their women undergo what is considered a straightforward operation of hysterectomy, tubal ligation, or laparoscopic excision of endometriosis in which the woman returns with severe incapacitating pelvic pain. The reason is not in the operative procedure that was uncomplicated, but it is difficult at times to persuade that to the woman involved. Possibly, there was a preexisting state that made this possible. In reviewing women presenting with postoperative onset of chronic pelvic pain, there is commonly a history of pain preceding the operation. This can take the form of severe dysmenorrhea, repetitive bouts of cystitis, or prior kidney stones. Pain causes chronic pain and while it is possible to generate chronic pelvic pain from an isolated procedure, it is much more common to see there was a previous pattern of repetitive pain. The shift to a chronic pain state might be identified as a risk with pain testing for sensitization.

Also, there is a troubling experience of undertaking an operative laparoscopy anticipating there is going to be endometriosis present and instead finding no disease whatsoever. Again, this leads to difficult explanations and often the patient will seek yet another laparoscopy.

These examples are fundamentally issues of pain and pain management. In order to have a strategy to inform these situations, pain testing might be of assistance.

Acknowledgements

The assistance of Drs. Giamberardino and Arendt-Nilesen are greatly appreciated. Funding was generously provided by The Canadian Institutes of Health Research.

Author details

John Jarrell
University of Calgary, Calgary, Alberta, Canada

*Address all correspondence to: jarrelljohnf@gmail.com

References

[1] Kuhlmann L, Olesen SS, Olesen AE, Arendt-Nielsen L, Drewes AM. Mechanism-based pain management in chronic pancreatitis—Is it time for a paradigm shift? Expert Review of Clinical Pharmacology. 2019;**12**(3):249-258

[2] Hellman KM, Roth GE, Dillane KE, Garrison EF, Oladosu FA, Clauw DJ, et al. Dysmenorrhea subtypes exhibit differential quantitative sensory assessment profiles. Pain. June 2020; **161**(6):1227-1236. DOI: 10.1097/j.pain.0000000000001826

[3] Grundstrom H, Gerdle B, Alehagen S, Bertero C, Arendt-Nielsen L, Kjolhede P. Reduced pain thresholds and signs of sensitization in women with persistent pelvic pain and suspected endometriosis. Acta Obstetricia et Gynecologica Scandinavica. 2019;**98**(3):327-336

[4] Bajaj P, Bajaj P, Madsen H, Arendt-Nielsen L. Endometriosis is associated with central sensitization: A psychophysical controlled study. The Journal of Pain. 2003;**4**(7):372-380

[5] Arendt-Nielsen L, Morlion B, Perrot S, Dahan A, Dickenson A, Kress HG, et al. Assessment and manifestation of central sensitisation across different chronic pain conditions. European Journal of Pain. 2018;**22**(2):216-241

[6] Mackenzie J. Symptoms and Their Interpretation. New York: Paul B. Hoeber; 1913

[7] Head H. On disturbances of sensation with special reference to the pain of visceral disease. Brain. 1893;**16**:133

[8] Giamberardino MA, Affaitati G, Fabrizio A, Costantini R. Myofascial pain syndromes and their evaluation. Best Practice & Research. Clinical Rheumatology. 2011;**25**(2):185-198

[9] Woolf CJ. Central sensitization: Implications for the diagnosis and treatment of pain. Pain. 2011;**152** (3 Suppl):S2-S15

[10] Yosef A, Allaire C, Williams C, Ahmed AG, Al-Hussaini T, Abdellah MS, et al. Multifactorial contributors to the severity of chronic pelvic pain in women. American Journal of Obstetrics and Gynecology. 2016;**215**(6): 760.e1-.e14

[11] Jarrell JV, Allaire G, Burgess C, Fortin S, Gerwin C, Lapensee R, et al. Consensus guidelines for the management of chronic pelvic pain. Journal of Obstetrics and Gynaecology. 2005;**29**(4):6

[12] Jarrell JV, Allaire G, Burgess C, Fortin S, Gerwin C, Lapensee R, et al. Consensus guidelines for the management of chronic pelvic pain. Journal of Obstetrics and Gynaecology. 2005;**27**(8):20

[13] Jarrell J, Giamberardino MA, Robert M, Nasr-Esfahani M. Bedside testing for chronic pelvic pain: Discriminating visceral from somatic pain. Pain Research and Treatment. 2011;**2011**:692102

[14] Nasr-Esfahani M, Jarrell J. Cotton-tipped applicator test: Validity and reliability in chronic pelvic pain. American Journal of Obstetrics and Gynecology. 2013;**208**(1):52 e1-5

[15] Jarrell JA-N, L. The negative laparoscopy unveiled. Journal of Endometriosis and Pelvic Pain Disorders. 2018;**10**(1):18-21

[16] Jarrell J, Robert M, Giamberardino MA, Tang S, Stephenson K. Pain, psychosocial tests,

pain sensitization and laparoscopic pelvic surgery. Scandinavian Journal of Pain. 2018;**18**(1):49-57

[17] Jarrell J. Gynecological pain, endometriosis, visceral disease, and the viscero-somatic connection. Journal of Musculoskeletal Pain. 2008;**16**(1-2):21

[18] Jarrell J. Diagnostic and operative laparoscopy in Alberta 1994-2006. Journal of Obstetrics and Gynaecology Canada. 2008;**30**(11):1045-1049

[19] Costello MF, Abbott J, Katz S, Vancaillie T, Wilson S. A prospective, randomized, double-blind, placebo-controlled trial of multimodal intraoperative analgesia for laparoscopic excision of endometriosis. Fertility and Sterility. 2010;**94**(2):436-443

[20] Sutton CJ, Ewen SP, Whitelaw N, Haines P. Prospective, randomized, double-blind, controlled trial of laser laparoscopy in the treatment of pelvic pain associated with minimal, mild, and moderate endometriosis. Fertility and Sterility. 1994;**62**(4):696-700

[21] Jarrell J, Mohindra R, Ross S, Taenzer P, Brant R. Laparoscopy and reported pain among patients with endometriosis. Journal of Obstetrics and Gynaecology Canada. 2005;**27**(5):477-485

[22] Jarrell J, Brant R, Leung W, Taenzer P. Women's pain experience predicts future surgery for pain associated with endometriosis. Journal of Obstetrics and Gynaecology Canada. 2007;**29**(12):988-991

Section 3

About Adenomyosis

Chapter 5

Adenomyosis

Wei Zheng and Boya Deng

Abstract

Adenomyosis is a benign uterus disease in which the invasion of the endometrial glands and/or stroma within myometrium is found and usually appears between the ages of 40 and 50 years in women. There are several differences in their pathogenesis. The secondary dysmenorrhea and menorrhagia are the common symptoms. Ultrasound sonography, MRI, CA125, and histological examination can be helpful for the diagnosis of adenomyosis. The treatment of adenomyosis depends on the patient's age, symptoms, and desire for future fertility, including medical treatment and surgical treatment.

Keywords: adenomyosis, hyperestrogenism, progesterone, laparoscopic, GnRHa, LNG-IUS

1. Introduction

Adenomyosis is a benign uterus disease in which the invasion of the endometrial glands and/or stroma within myometrium is found and usually appears between the ages of 40 and 50 years in women [1]. It can result in debilitating pelvic pain, abnormal uterine bleeding, and infertility. It was first described in 1860 by Rokitansky, and in 1896, Cullen suggested the term "adenomyosis." Adenomyosis is an estrogen-dependent disease similar to endometriosis and it regresses rapidly after the menopause. However, adenomyosis is a poorly understood gynecologic disease.

2. Prevalence

Most cases of adenomyosis were discovered in multiparous women during the transitional years (40–50 years). Women of age range 30–60 years also can be affected. The incidence of adenomyosis remains unknown, because the disease is usually recorded on the base of hospital and surgical reports, it is generally estimated that 20% of women have adenomyosis. However, an analysis of multiple myometrial sections may reveal an incidence as high as 65% [2].

3. Pathogenesis

Endometriosis and adenomyosis are closely linked diseases, but there are several differences in their pathogenesis. Four theories have been proposed to explain adenomyosis: heredity, trauma, hyperketonemia, and viral transmission. Although the exact cause is unknown, the most widely accepted theory of histogenesis was proposed by Meyer in 1900. Meyer postulated that the normal barrier between

IntechOpen

the endometrium and myometrium is somehow attenuated. The most held theory regarding adenomyosis is the endometrial basalis layer invades through the end myometrial junctional zone (JZ) into the myometrium after trauma on the endometrium [3]. Estrogen and progesterone likely play a role in its development after invagination of the endometrium. Another theory is that adenomyosis is caused by metaplasia of the Müllerian tissue [4]. Ren et al. demonstrated that Belin 1 expression was decreased in eutopic endometrium, and negatively correlated with serum CA125 and pelvic pain. Belin 1, therefore, may play a role in the pathogenesis and progression of adenomyosis [5]. The tissue injury and repair (TIAR) mechanism is activated in response to tissue auto-traumatization. This mechanism leads to a specific physiological process that promoted local production of Bcl-2, and plays an important role in the occurrence and development of adenomyosis [6]. The levels of anti-smooth muscle antibody positive and collage I positive myofibroblasts are significantly higher in the JZ of women with adenomyosis than in those without [3], as the evidence of tissue microtrauma and activation of the TIAR mechanism.

Hyperestrogenism is suggested to result from increased local aromatization, and decreased local estrogen metabolism in the eutopic and ectopic endometrium of patients with adenomyosis. Hyperestrogenism may promote elevated mechanical strains and stresses that could injure cells in the junctional zone (JZ) [7, 8].

Recently, studies of embryonic pluripotent Müllerian remnants and differentiation of adult stem cells have also been reported [4, 9, 10]. Epithelial-mesenchymal transition (EMT) is biological process involved in embryological development, tissue repair, and cancer cell migration, but the mechanism triggering EMT in adenomyosis has not yet been elucidated [11].

4. Pathology

There are two types of adenomyosis: focal and diffuse. The typical uterus with adenomyosis is enlarged compared to normal ones. The thickening of the uterine

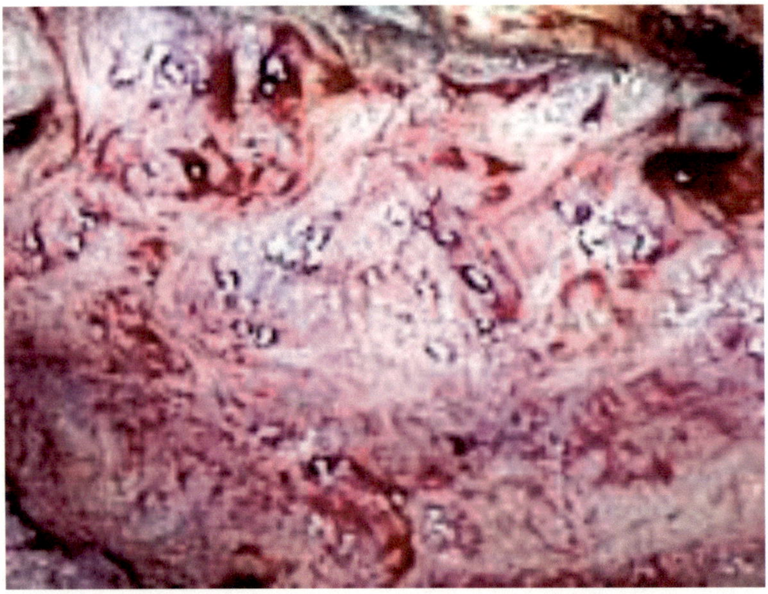

Figure 1.
The thickening of the uterine well is made up of trabeculated areas, stippled or granular in appearance, with small yellow or darker cystic tissues which contain serous fluid or stale blood.

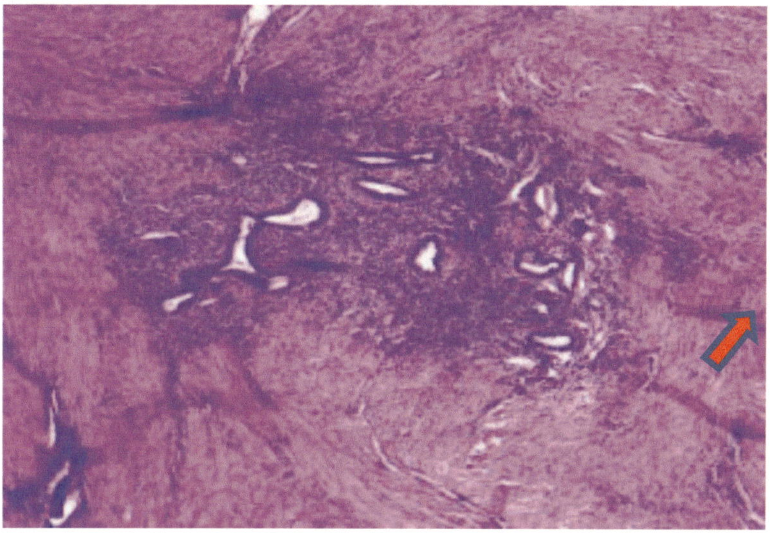

Figure 2.
The presence of endometrial tissue, glands and stroma are within the myometrium.

wall was made up of focal or diffused adenomyosis areas stippled or granular in appearance, with darker cystic lesions that may contain serous fluid or stale hemorrhage (**Figure 1**); in some rare cases, adenomyosis may present as a large chocolate cyst (cystic adenomyosis) [12].

The microscopic feature of adenomyosis is the presence of endometrial tissue including glands and stroma cells within the myometrium (**Figure 2**).

More than 80% of women with adenomyosis have some pathological process in the uterus. Patients have associated leiomyomas [13] and endometriosis [14].

5. Symptoms

Early adenomyosis is asymptomatic, only about one-third of women with adenomyosis have symptoms. Secondary dysmenorrhea and menorrhagia are the common symptoms. The severity of dysmenorrhea correlates with the increasing number of invasions. It is thought to be caused by increased prostaglandin production found in adenomyosis tissues compared with normal myometrium. Approximately 60% of women suffer from abnormal uterine bleeding; menorrhagia and dysmenorrhea are the two major adenomyosis-associated symptoms, and 30% of patients with these symptoms have typical secondary, progressive dysmenorrhea [15]. Menorrhagia with adenomyosis includes excessively heavy or prolonged menstrual bleeding. Some patients' symptoms are not common but may include menstrual irregularities. Some patients with adenomyosis have the history of infertility or abortion.

6. Diagnosis

6.1 Ultrasound sonography

Imaging with transvaginal ultrasound (TVUS) can identify the subtle myometrial changes of adenomyosis, the findings may include: (1) the anterior or posterior myometrial wall appearing thicker, (2) small myometrial hypoechoic cysts, (3) endometrium JZ extending into the myometrium, (4) appearance of focal adenomyosis as discrete hypoechoic nodules that may be differentiated from leiomyoma by poorly defined margins, and (5) myometrial hyperplasia. Three-dimensional transvaginal ultrasonography can improve the diagnostic accuracy with variable ranges of sensitivity between 70 and 93% and specificity between 86 and 93% for diagnosing adenomyosis by TVUS [16].

6.2 MRI

MRI has been shown to be highly accurate in the diagnosis of adenomyosis.
It can differentiate between adenomyosis and the fibroids. MR imaging may be complimentary (**Figure 3**). The main MRI criterion for diagnosing adenomyosis is by detection of high-intensity tiny myometrial cysts in the inner myometrium, irregularity, and asymmetric junctional zone. MRI can distinguish the subtypes of adenomyosis: diffuse and solid or cystic adenomyoma.

6.3 CA-125

There are studies find the levels of the ovarian epithelial tumor antigen CA-125 patients with adenomyosis might be high. After the therapy, it might decrease.

6.4 Histological examination

The gold standard for the diagnosis of adenomyosis is histological examination. The diagnosis is usually based on histologic findings in surgical specimens after hysterectomy.

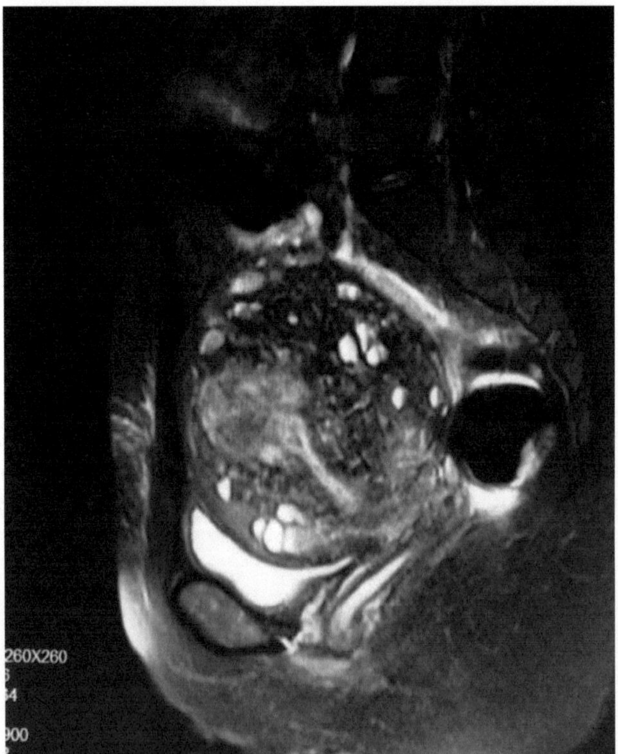

Figure 3.
MRI of adenomyosis.

7. Treatment

The treatment of adenomyosis depends on the patient's age, symptoms, and desire for fertility.

7.1 Medical treatment

7.1.1 GnRHa

Gonadotropin-releasing hormone (GnRH) agonists have been shown to release pain and reduce the adenomyotic lesions' size [17].

GnRHa agonists cause hypoestrogenism, resulting in adverse effects such as hot flashes, vaginal dryness, and bone mineral loss.

7.1.2 Oral dienogest

Dienogest, a novel 19-nortestosterone derivative, is a synthetic oral progestin that is highly selective for progesterone receptors. Dienogest reduces the painful symptoms in women with endometriosis [18].

A recent study of the oral dienogest for premenopausal menorrhagia and pelvic pains in women with uterine adenomyosis indicated that oral dienogest might be a valuable alternative for treatment of premenopausal pelvic pains in women with uterine adenomyosis [19]. Another pilot study presented the results on the efficacy and safety of dienogest in the treatment of symptomatic adenomyosis. Dienogest significantly reduced adenomyosis-associated pelvic pain as well as serum CA-125 and CA 19-9 levels [20].

7.1.3 LNG-IUS

Menorrhagia associated with adenomyosis can be treated with levonorgestrel-releasing IUS that releases levonorgestrel, 20 μg/day. It is placed in uterus within 7 days of menstruation.

7.1.4 Other drugs

Danazol has been the medical therapy for treatment of adenomyosis for several years. Danazol has a direct antiestrogen effect on endometriotic lesions

Nonsteroidal anti-inflammatory drugs (NSAIDs) can relieve mild pain associated with adenomyosis. NSAIDs are the analgesia and anti-inflammatory agents through the pathway of inhibition of PGE2 and COX-2.

Combination oral contraceptives can be used to induce endometrial atrophy and decrease endometrial prostaglandin production to improve dysmenorrhea and menorrhagia.

7.2 Surgical treatment

7.2.1 Hysterectomy

This is the definitive treatment of adenomyosis; however, most of the patients do not accept the surgery of total hysterectomy, with or without ovarian conservation. Patients who have a desire for pregnancy can be treated by focal adenomyosis resection using either laparotomy or laparoscopic surgery.

7.2.2 Ablation of adenomyosis using high-intensity focused ultrasound (HIFU)

High-intensity focused ultrasound (HIFU) ablation, which was initially developed for the treatment of solid tumors, is now successfully implemented in the treatment of uterine fibroids and adenomyosis [21–23]. Several prospective studies have demonstrated ranges of effectivity between 81 and 87% [21–24]. After HIFU therapy, MRI showed the diffuse adenomyosis in **Figure 4(a)** and the nonperfused area of the lesion without damage to the surrounding normal tissue in **Figure 4(b)**. Rarely serious complications including major permanent injuries were observed. Ultrasound-guided HIFU ablation may be a safe and effective noninvasive alternative in the treatment of symptomatic adenomyosis.

7.2.3 Ablation of endometrium with adenomyosis using MEA or NovaSure

Endometrial ablation or resection using hysteroscopy has been used to successfully treat dysmenorrhea and menorrhagia caused by adenomyosis. But it is not acceptable if future pregnancy desired.

7.2.4 Uterine artery embolization (UAE)

It has been used to relieve symptoms for adenomyosis. UAE has favorable outcomes in symptomatic adenomyosis, both short-term and long-term [25]. Due to the limited clinical data, the side effects on ovarian function and future pregnancy after UAE are still not clear.

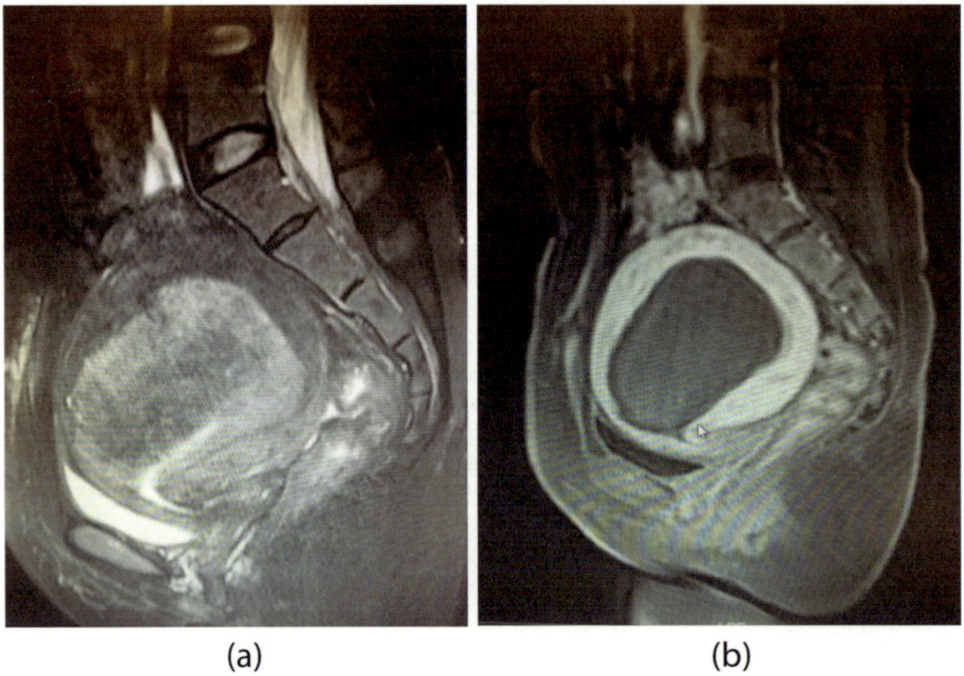

Figure 4.
MRI of adenomyosis in (a) showed the diffuse lesion before HIFU, and (b) showed the nonperfused area of the lesion without damage to the surrounding normal tissue after HIFU.

8. Adenomyosis malignant transformation

As with other pathologies of endometriosis, adenomyosis may goes malignant transformation. It is not clear whether some malignancies being as such or progress from benign disease to malignant. The neoplasia arises coincidentally in continuity with endometriotic implants.

Although adenomyosis is usually benign, it might also be a precursor of malignant disease. As the incidence of adenomyosis malignant transformation is low, and its clinical manifestation is nonspecific, it may only be confirmed by postoperative pathological examination. Malignant neoplasia occurs rarely in the glands and/or stroma; these tumors may be in the form of adenocarcinomas, sarcomas, or carcinosarcomas. Further investigations with large samples may provide additional data of the prognosis of adenomyosis malignant transformation [26]. Some of the risk factors of malignant adenomyosis include age between 40 and 50 years, early menarche, short menstrual cycle, first delivery at young age, fertility, curettage during early trimester of pregnancy, obesity, and history of tamoxifen intake. The expression of both PR and ER was positive in patients with endometrial carcinoma combined with adenomyosis or endometrial carcinoma combined with uterine fibroids, and the expression of p53 and Ki67 was positive in eutopic malignant endometrium and negative in normal ectopic endometrium, which may provide additional pathological data on adenomyosis malignant transformation [26, 27].

9. Conclusion

Adenomyosis is a condition in which the inner lining of the uterus (the endometrial) breaks through the uterus myometrium. Adenomyosis can cause menstrual cramps, lower abdominal pain, and heavy periods, and negatively impact on a woman's quality of life. The condition can be located throughout the entire endometrium or localized in one spot. Nonsteroidal anti-inflammatory drugs (NSAIDs) can relieve mild pain associated with adenomyosis. Symptoms such as heavy or painful periods can be controlled with hormonal therapies. HIFU focused on a small focal region to increase tissue temperature sufficiently, which causes irreparable cell damage in the target adenomyosis lesions at a certain depth. And uterine artery embolization, the minimally invasive procedure, used to block the blood vessels therefore causes adenomyosis shrinks. Endometrial ablation destroys the lining of the uterus and relief from the heavy bleeding. The only definitive cure for adenomyosis is a hysterectomy.

Acknowledgements

Thanks to Dr. Courtney Marsh, his book "Endometriosis" is an influential reference in organizing our paper.

Author details

Wei Zheng* and Boya Deng
Department of Gynecology, The Second Affiliated Hospital, School of Medicine, Zhejiang University, Hangzhou, Zhejiang Province, China

*Address all correspondence to: zhengwei@zju.edu.cn

References

[1] McElin TW, Bird CC. Adenomyosis of the uterus. Obstetrics and Gynecology Annual. 1974;**3**(0): 425-441

[2] Devlieger R, D'Hooghe T, Timmerman D. Uterine adenomyosis in the infertility clinic. Human Reproduction Update. 2003;**9**(2): 139-147

[3] Ibrahim MG et al. Myofibroblasts are evidence of chronic tissue microtrauma at the endometrial-myometrial junctional zone in uteri with adenomyosis. Reproductive Sciences. 2017;**24**(10):1410-1418

[4] Vannuccini S et al. Pathogenesis of adenomyosis: An update on molecular mechanisms. Reproductive Biomedicine Online. 2017;**35**(5):592-601

[5] Ren Y et al. Decreased expression of Beclin 1 in eutopic endometrium of women with adenomyosis. Archives of Gynecology and Obstetrics. 2010;**282**(4):401-406

[6] Li J et al. The expression of Bcl-2 in adenomyosis and its effect on proliferation, migration, and apoptosis of endometrial stromal cells. Pathology, Research and Practice. 2019;**215**(8):152477

[7] Leyendecker G, Wildt L, Mall G. The pathophysiology of endometriosis and adenomyosis: Tissue injury and repair. Archives of Gynecology and Obstetrics. 2009;**280**(4):529-538

[8] Leyendecker G, Wildt L. A new concept of endometriosis and adenomyosis: Tissue injury and repair (TIAR). Hormone Molecular Biology and Clinical Investigation. 2011;**5**(2):125-142

[9] Chan RW, Schwab KE, Gargett CE. Clonogenicity of human endometrial epithelial and stromal cells. Biology of Reproduction. 2004;**70**(6):1738-1750

[10] Gargett CE, Schwab KE, Deane JA. Endometrial stem/progenitor cells: The first 10 years. Human Reproduction Update. 2016;**22**(2):137-163

[11] Chen YJ et al. Oestrogen-induced epithelial-mesenchymal transition of endometrial epithelial cells contributes to the development of adenomyosis. The Journal of Pathology. 2010;**222**(3):261-270

[12] Chapron C et al. Relationship between the magnetic resonance imaging appearance of adenomyosis and endometriosis phenotypes. Human Reproduction. 2017;**32**(7):1393-1401

[13] Brucker SY et al. Clinical characteristics indicating adenomyosis coexisting with leiomyomas: A retrospective, questionnaire-based study. Fertility and Sterility. 2014;**101**(1):237-241.e1

[14] Di Donato N et al. Prevalence of adenomyosis in women undergoing surgery for endometriosis. European Journal of Obstetrics, Gynecology, and Reproductive Biology. 2014;**181**:289-293

[15] Garcia L, Isaacson K. Adenomyosis: Review of the literature. Journal of Minimally Invasive Gynecology. 2011;**18**(4):428-437

[16] Rasmussen CK, Hansen ES, Dueholm M. Inter-rater agreement in the diagnosis of adenomyosis by 2- and 3-dimensional transvaginal ultrasonography. Journal of Ultrasound in Medicine. 2019;**38**(3):657-666

[17] Nelson JR, Corson SL. Long-term management of adenomyosis with a gonadotropin-releasing hormone agonist: A case report. Fertility and Sterility. 1993;**59**(2):441-443

[18] Gordts S, Grimbizis G, Campo R. Symptoms and classification of uterine adenomyosis, including the place of hysteroscopy in diagnosis. Fertility and Sterility. 2018;**109**(3):380-388.e1

[19] Harada T et al. Dienogest is as effective as intranasal buserelin acetate for the relief of pain symptoms associated with endometriosis--a randomized, double-blind, multicenter, controlled trial. Fertility and Sterility. 2009;**91**(3):675-681

[20] Fawzy M, Mesbah Y. Comparison of dienogest versus triptorelin acetate in premenopausal women with adenomyosis: A prospective clinical trial. Archives of Gynecology and Obstetrics. 2015;**292**(6):1267-1271

[21] Liu X et al. Clinical predictors of long-term success in ultrasound-guided high-intensity focused ultrasound ablation treatment for adenomyosis: A retrospective study. Medicine. 2016;**95**(3):e2443

[22] Fan TY et al. Feasibility of MRI-guided high intensity focused ultrasound treatment for adenomyosis. European Journal of Radiology. 2012;**81**(11):3624-3630

[23] Zhou M et al. Ultrasound-guided high-intensity focused ultrasound ablation for adenomyosis: The clinical experience of a single center. Fertility and Sterility. 2011;**95**(3):900-905

[24] Guo Q et al. High intensity focused ultrasound treatment of adenomyosis: A comparative study. International Journal of Hyperthermia. 2018;**35**(1):505-509

[25] de Bruijn AM et al. Uterine artery embolization for the treatment of adenomyosis: A systematic review and meta-analysis. Journal of Vascular and Interventional Radiology. 2017;**28**(12):1629-1642.e1

[26] Mao X, Zheng W, Mao W. Malignant changes in adenomyosis in patients with endometrial adenocarcinoma: A case series. Medicine. 2017;**96**(43):e8336

[27] Sasaki T et al. Endometrioid adenocarcinoma arising from adenomyosis: Report and immunohistochemical analysis of an unusual case. Pathology International. 2001;**51**(4):308-313

Section 4

Endometriosis and Infertility

Chapter 6

Benefits of Surgical Intervention in Women with Endometriosis-Related Infertility

Popov Alexander, Koval Alexey, Fedorov Anton, Tyurina Svetlana, Fedotova Irina and Khabibullakh Tamana

Abstract

Endometriosis is one of the most common gynecological diseases in the world with a great variety of symptoms and clinical features. The true prevalence rates in the general population are not known, but according to different authors, endometriosis is to be found in 10% in women of reproductive age. According to different publications, around half of the patients with infertility were diagnosed with endometriosis which change the significance of this disease from the only female to a socio-economical problem. In this chapter, we will focus on the current view on endometriosis-associated infertility, from superficial to adenomyosis, with a closer view of surgical treatment, as it is still the standard of care for diagnosis and in severe cases—treatment of the disease.

Keywords: adenomyosis, DIE, deep infiltrative endometriosis, endometrioma, peritoneal endometriosis, infertility, IVF

1. Introduction

Today, the medical community considers endometriosis as a significant disease and problem. According to different resources, about 176 million women are suffering from the disease worldwide. In multination, multicenter study [1] about 50% of gynecologists polled in Russia in 2007 examined 7–28 patients with endometriosis per month (240 patients per year). The number was almost equal to that of patients with myoma.

Endometriosis is known to be found in 60% of women aged under 30. More important is the fact that there is a 7-year delay from the first disease manifestation to the diagnosis [2].

The physician should suspect the endometriosis if the following complaints are present [3]:

- Dysmenorrhea, acyclic pelvic pain, deep dyspareunia, and infertility
- If a woman of reproductive age has the following symptoms: dyschesia, dysuria, hematuria, and rectorrhagia

Even though the exact mechanism of endometriosis-associated infertility is still unknown, some aspects are well studied. Endometriosis has an influence on the quality of peritoneal fluid with growing macrophage concentration as well as proteases and cytokines negatively influencing the quality of oocytes, sperm, embryo, and fallopian tube potential.

It is difficult to recommend the optimal treatment as the development of the disease is unpredictable—from asymptomatic to very aggressive though pelvic pain and infertility usually called "active endometriosis" [4].

The American Society of Reproductive Medicine (ASRM) classification of endometriosis describes four stages of the disease. But that does not always correlate with the actual symptoms (pain, infertility, etc.) [5–7]. The more you work with this classification, the more it becomes obvious that patients with the same stages of the disease by ASRM classification, in fact, are incomparable. The ideal approach to endometriosis treatment should take into consideration how active the disease is. The "active" disease requires a combined treatment. The combination of surgical, hormonal treatment, and in vitro fertilization (IVF) could be individually chosen in each specific case of infertile patients.

For an easier understanding of how to treat endometriosis-associated infertility, it is better to separate the disease in four different phenotypes: superficial, endometrioma, deep infiltrated endometriosis, and adenomyosis.

2. Superficial endometriosis

The "gold" standard of superficial endometriosis treatment is laparoscopy. The common indications for surgery are pelvic pains and infertility. Hysteroscopy and biopsy, laparoscopy with fallopian tube perturbation, adhesiolysis, endometriosis staging with ablation, and/or removal lesions could be recommended. Pregnancy rate (PR) after laparoscopic treatment is the same for all stages [5].

However, if pelvic pain dominates, empirical conservative medical treatment could be applied. Infertile patients should be informed of alternative methods of treatment. Pregnancy can be achieved with IVF without surgery.

Laparoscopic treatment of minimal and mild endometriotic lesions (stage 1 and 2 ASRM) is justified in the case of pelvic pain because their destruction significantly decreases the pain compared with diagnostic laparoscopy alone. In this context, ablation and excision give identical results in terms of pain reduction. It is not recommended to treat asymptomatic patients. Literature shows no interest in uterine nerve ablation in case of dysmenorrhea due to minimal and mild endometriosis. With regard to treatment of minimal and mild endometriosis in infertile patients, only two studies can be selected, and both show that laparoscopy with excision or ablation and ablation of adhesions is superior to diagnostic laparoscopy alone also in terms of pregnancy rate [8].

The effectiveness of adjuvant hormonal treatment after surgery is not improved. Most hormonal medications have a contraceptive effect and make spontaneous pregnancy almost impossible.

IVF should be recommended in cases of fallopian tubes' low potential and/or male infertility. The spontaneous PR is very low if there are several simultaneous infertility factors. The very important factor is also the maternal age. At present, there is no generally accepted age for patients who should be recommended to go straight to ART after surgery and who could try to achieve spontaneous pregnancy. But a lot of surgeons agree that the maternal age of 35 and higher should be considered in favor of ART after surgery.

de Ziegler's et al. in the review [9] presented an algorithm for the management of infertility associated with endometriosis. This algorithm is presented in **Figure 1**.

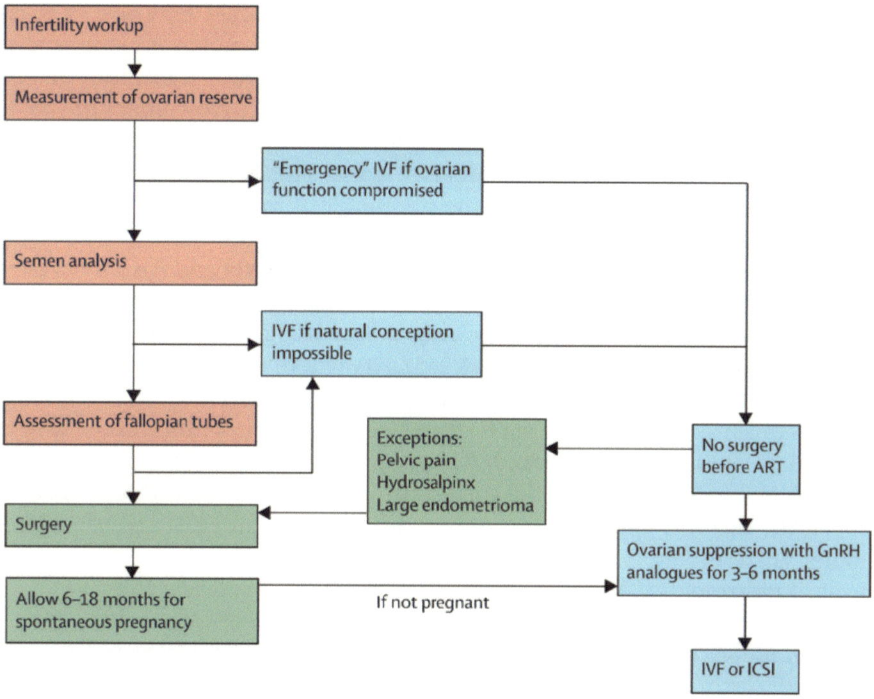

Figure 1.
Algorithm for management of infertility associated with endometriosis [9]. IVF, in vitro fertilization; ART, assisted reproductive technologies; GnRH, gonadotropin-releasing hormone; ICSI, intracytoplasmic sperm injection.

The repeated surgery is not recommended due to low spontaneous PR. The second (third, fourth, etc.) laparoscopy results in further IVF. This is not because of the bad surgery performed but because endometriosis is a chronical complex disease, which is associated with pelvic inflammation and profound alterations of peritoneal fluid, which surrounds the pelvic organs [10]. These alterations could affect natural conception.

3. Deep infiltrating endometriosis

Recently, the number of patients with deep infiltrating endometriosis (DIE) has been steadily increasing. It is estimated to affect up to 12% of all women with endometriosis. DIE is detected in 50–70% of patients of reproductive period with pain syndrome. This disease is diagnosed when there is an infiltration of 5 mm or more beneath the peritoneal surface [11] and/or an involvement of muscular layer of affected organ into the pathologic process is found [12].

DIE is characterized by multifocal distribution with the involvement of peritoneum, pelvic spaces, uterus ligaments, rectovaginal septum, vagina, intestine, bowel, ureters and bladder, and diaphragm. The feature of such dissemination is the lymphovascular invasion, the degree of which one is correlated with sizes of the primary endometrioid nodules. It is also estimated that endometriotic lesions seem to infiltrate the bowel wall preferentially along the nerves, even at distance from palpated nodules, while the mucosa is rarely and only focally involved [13].

There is no correlation between the stage of endometriosis, how deep it is, the number of symptoms, and their duration. Infertility is the most frequent symptom. Development of infertility in DIE is multifactorial: pelvic adhesions, the decrease in ovarian reserve, and a poor quality of oocytes in case of involvement of the ovaries. It is assumed that changes in ectopic endometrium are not as pronounced in patients with DIE as in cases of severe adenomyosis. This conclusion could be made on the basis that in patients with DIE, the frequency of miscarriages is less, and the frequency of successful IVF attempts is satisfactory.

In cases of lesions difficult location (myometrium, bowel and ileum, pararectal space), where removal is technically impossible or highly risky, the combination of surgery and medication is very promising. According to the data of Darai et al., spontaneous PR after surgical treatment is 51.1%, whereas IVF PR is 18.9% [14].

The medical treatment of deep infiltrating endometriosis may decrease symptoms and is often associated with such side effects as noncyclic bleedings, weight increase, libido loss, and headaches. It doesn't provide the control of disease course in a long-term period, and when the treatment is over, the disease progresses. Moreover, the medical options have contraceptive effects and can't be used when pregnancy is attempted [15].

Surgical treatment of DIE and infertility in most cases is preferable. Spontaneous pregnancy rate (PR) after surgical treatment of DIE is close to 50% [15]. It means that every second patient with DIE and infertility will not require IVF.

At the same time, we must not forget that the rate of severe postoperative complications of DIE treatment (rectal bleeding, anastomosis insufficiency, rectovaginal fistulas, abscesses, fecal peritonitis) is 10% [16]. Patients must be informed about the possible complications and results of DIE infertility treatment. IVF is preferable if other symptoms (pain, dyspareunia, dyschezia, low urinary tract symptoms) are absent.

There are no doubts about the removal of such endometriotic nodules in the bladder and parametrium, but the choice of ideal surgical approach to the treatment of bowel endometriosis is more controversial. Three types of surgical removal of endometrioid nodules are described: shaving, discoid, and bowel resection. According to the data of Abrao et al. [17], the treatment algorithm for deep endometriosis compromising the bowel must be individualized (**Figure 2**). "Conservative" surgery (shaving) is more appropriate in reproductive medicine due to its less risk. Surgery of DIE including bowel resection should be considered as a second-line treatment after failed IVF and in cases when there is a presentation of such symptoms as pelvic pain, dyspareunia, dyschezia, and bowel stenosis.

We can't recommend the anticipating spontaneous pregnancy after surgery for more than 9–12 months. It is attended with the risk of recurrent endometriosis and pelvic pain, which will make IVF more complicated.

In Malzoni et al. [18] publication, indications for radical colorectal surgery are described and clearly stated. Absolute indications are severe pain, bowel stenosis with functional organ compromise, and infertility in patients after unsuccessful IVF attempts even asymptomatic. The relative indications to radical surgery are the following: infertility in young patients (<35 years), infertility (even aged >35 years) after two or more IVF failures before the oocyte donation, and increased risks of pregnancy and delivery complications.

The last indication is one of the most disputable. Exacoustos et al. [19] described the obstetrical complication in patients with colorectal endometriosis. The number of premature delivery <37 weeks was five times more in colorectal endometriosis group than the control group. Placenta previa was diagnosed in every six patients with posterior endometriosis (only 1 case from 300 patients in control group).

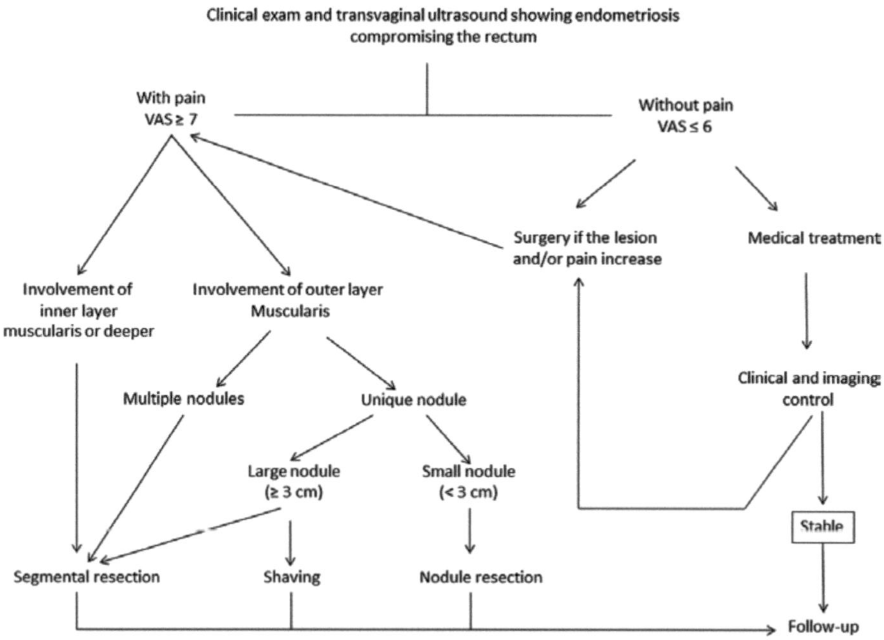

Figure 2.
Treatment algorithm for deep endometriosis compromising the bowel by Abrao et al. [17] (VAS—visual analog scale).

Cesarian section was performed in 68.3% in colorectal endometriosis group. Hysterectomy, hemoperitoneum, bowel resection, and bladder injury were described in 3.6–7.1% of patients with colorectal endometriosis.

The pathogenic mechanisms of pregnancy complications can be the following: endometriosis-related chronic inflammation, adhesions and their mechanical implications, and invasion of decidualized ectopic endometrium to the vessel walls.

Taking into account the risks of surgical intervention in cases of DIE, it's reasonable to perform the operation in the specialized medical centers by multidisciplinary team, including gynecologist, urologist, colorectal surgeon, and fertility specialist. But endometriosis is a gynecological disease, and the gynecologist should be the leader of this team.

A very important practical question is what would be the recommendations if an unexperienced surgeon found DIE with diagnostic laparoscopy? In such case no one has repealed one of the basic rules of medical practice—"primum non nocere"—do not harm. If the surgeon is not enough experienced, to prevent complications, it would be better to stop the surgery after doing those steps, which could be done, according to the experience and send the patient to the clinic, which is focused on DIE treatment. Providing all the information about the presence of the disease to the patient is essential.

4. Endometrioma

In recent years, indications for surgical treatment of endometriomas in infertile patients are reconsidered due to the negative impact of surgery on the ovarian reserve, especially in recurrent cysts and bilateral localization. The surgeon faces the question which patients should be operated and if expectant management is chosen and then what period is appropriate. Comparative evaluation of cystectomy of non-endometriotic cyst (dermoid, serous, and mucinous cystadenoma) and endometriomas highlighted that some ovarian tissue was removed only in 6% during surgical treatment of non-endometriotic cysts. In contrast, in the resection of endometriomas, ovarian tissue was present in the specimen in 54% of cases [1].

Nowadays, there is no consensus on the size of endometriomas which should be treated surgically. International recommendations indicate surgical treatment for cysts larger than 3–4 cm [3, 20] and according to some other guidelines, more than 6 cm.

According to some published data, surgery on the ovaries before IVF does not improve reproductive outcomes. The exception is large endometriomas which are difficult to puncture [21]. Asymptomatic endometriotic cysts of small size do not require surgical treatment, especially in patients older than 35 years. Surgical treatment must be performed in patients with long-term infertility in the presence of cysts greater than 4 cm [3].

In patients with a high risk of ovarian reserve damage (second ovarian surgery, bilateral localization, late reproductive age), it is necessary to consider cryopreservation of embryos or vitrification of oocyte before surgical treatment.

Surgical treatment can be performed in three ways—aspiration, sclerotherapy, and laparoscopic/open removal. The endometriotic lining of endometrioma may undergo pressure atrophy, and that spontaneous resolution of cyst can be achieved by simple aspiration by ultrasound or laparoscopic control. In difficult cases (adhesions, high risks of anesthesia, recurrence of small endometrioma), transvaginal puncture by ultrasound guidance could be recommended. According to different publications, the recurrence rate for sclerotherapy is 9.1–66.7% and could be decreased to 12% by the use of 95% ethanol in situ [22]. However, this procedure has been associated with postoperative pelvic abscesses.

If the surgery is to be performed, then the "gold" standard in case of endometrioma and infertility is laparoscopic cystectomy. Cystectomy can be performed in two ways: cyst ablation and enucleation. Laparoscopic cystectomy demonstrates the best results in achieving pregnancy for the first identified unilateral endometriomas. The spontaneous PR after cystectomy is more than 60%.

However, in the second surgery, partial capsule removal and ablation are the better options (to save ovarian reserve). In case of bilateral endometriomas in more advanced reproductive age and recurrent endometrioma, urgent IVF is indicated (the risk of decreased ovarian reserve). The removal of small endometrioma does not have an impact on cumulative PR. In some cases (recurrent endometrioma, difficulty in follicle puncture), sclerotherapy by ultrasound control could be recommended.

There are pitfalls of endometrioma's surgery. Surgery should be performed in the follicular phase to prevent recurrence. High power electrosurgical technique should be avoided. Bipolar coagulation (max 30 Watts) and/or suturing of the ovarian tissue is safer. Ablation can be applied for recurrence endometrioma in particular. New energies (PlasmaJet, CO_2 laser, argon-spread).

In our unpublished study, from 2010 to 2018, we performed 1187 laparoscopic procedures with removing of endometriomas in Moscow Regional Scientific Research Institute of Obstetrics and Gynecology. The average age of patients was 31.6 years old. Among them we make a follow up in 530 patients, and only 259 were included in the study. From 259 patients 105 have primary infertility before surgery (40.5%), 45 (17.37%) have secondary infertility, and 93 (35.9%) did not desire a pregnancy. In total, infertility was detected in 150 cases (57.9%). Laparoscopy and cyst removal (stripping) were done in the majority of cases—211 (81.6%); in 48 (18.4%) ovarium resection with the cyst was performed. Spontaneous pregnancy was registered among 77 women (51.3%). In 16 cases pregnancy was unexpected. Twenty-eight patients (18.6%) became pregnant after IVF. Cumulative pregnancy rate was 70% (105 patients). Ineffective attempts of spontaneous conception were

30, and IVF attempts were also unsuccessful in 36 cases (24%). After surgery, hormonal therapy was prescribed: dienogest in 34.3%, COC in 15%, and gonadotropin-releasing hormone agonists (GnRH-a) in 1.9% cases. The recurrence rate of the disease was 13.1% (34 cases).

There are the risks of nonsurgical management of patients with cysts and infertility [23]. The conditions with an expected high risk of complications, if patients go to IVF without surgical treatment, are the following: low ovarian responsiveness to the stimulation, low quality of oocytes, technical difficulties for ovarian puncture, endometrioma rupture, injury to adjacent organs, infection of the endometrioma, follicular fluid contamination, progression of endometriosis, pregnancy complications, the opportunity to miss the malignancy, and/or cancer development after IVF.

However, the meaning of surgery was overestimated. Surgical treatment did not improve an ovarian responsiveness to the stimulation, quality of oocytes, rate of technical difficulties during ovarian puncture, rate of injury to adjacent organs during this procedure, follicular fluid contamination, progression of endometriosis, and pregnancy complication rate.

5. Adenomyosis and infertility

Adenomyosis is a common gynecological disease, defined as the presence of ectopic endometrial epithelium and stroma in the myometrium.

Through the twentieth century before the widespread of transvaginal ultrasound (TVU) and magnetic resonance imaging (MRI) techniques, adenomyosis remained the disease, whose diagnosis was based on histological examination of the specimen after hysterectomy. As this examination was held after the surgery, the connection between infertility and adenomyosis was not well established. However, over the last three decades, the introduction of new diagnostic tools, mentioned above (TVU and MRI), made it possible to study adenomyosis without performing surgery. The measuring of the inner myometrium or myometrial junctional zone (JZ) described by Hricak group [24], provided new noninvasive diagnostic criteria for adenomyosis [25]. These new diagnostic tools allow us to diagnose the adenomyosis from early to advanced stages and see the progressing of the disease with high sensitivity and specificity. By different authors, the sensitivity and specificity range is 53–89% and 65–98% respectively. Although there is a great success in noninvasive diagnosis, the real incidence of adenomyosis is still unknown. The prevalence has been reported to range from 1 to 70%. This large range primarily reflects the lack of agreed diagnostic standards both by imaging tools and pathological analyses.

Even though many classifications, as well as scoring systems, have been proposed since the first mentioning of endometriosis as a disease, no widespread agreement on a classification for endometriosis has been reached. Unfortunately, there is no ideal classification of endometriosis that would be able to reflect all the aspects of the disease, the pathogenesis, anatomical distribution, clinical manifestation, progression, and recurrence.

The clinical presentation of adenomyosis can vary from patient to patient, but the main symptoms are abnormal uterine bleeding and dysmenorrhea, occurring in approximately 65% of patients [26]. Today there is a strong data that there is a correlation between the type, localization, and the number of endometriotic lesions and painful symptoms [27]. Despite the fact that the link between infertility and adenomyosis is still a subject of debate, the association between these two processes is clinically recognized [28]. Infertility is found in 11–12% of patients with adenomyosis [29].

The effect of adenomyosis on fertility has been assessed by examining its prevalence in infertility in patients or its effect on the outcomes of assisted reproduction technologies (ART). In a review by Campo et al. [30], several pathogenesis hypotheses of infertility in patients with adenomyosis are described. The first one was proposed by Kunz et al. [31, 32], which points out the idea of thickening and disruption of the myometrial JZ which can result in perturbed uterine peristalsis. In 1984 Birnholz [33] has published his data about the presence of contraction waves in the myometrium: using transabdominal ultrasound, he showed that uterine peristaltic activity originates exclusively from the JZ, while the outer myometrium remains static. During the follicular and periovulatory phases, contraction waves have a cervico-fundal orientation, and their amplitude and frequency increase significantly towards the time of ovulation. There is an idea that adenomyosis causes infertility by impairing sperm transport.

The second hypothesis is focused on biochemical and functional alterations in both eutopic and heterotopic endometrium in individuals with adenomyosis [34]. These alterations could lead to lower receptivity, as suggested by the presence of "implantation marker" defects. This increased knowledge has created new therapeutic options, including the block of local aromatase production through the use of selective estrogen receptor modulators, estrogen-progestin combinations, and gonadotropin-releasing hormone super agonists.

The third hypothesis proposes that the presence of an abnormal concentration of intrauterine free radicals [35] and of altered decidualization [36] is also suggestive of altered receptivity. The authors propose that free radicals may adversely affect eggs and fertilized eggs in adenomyosis by a similar mechanism to that in endometriosis. The exaggerated expression of these enzymes suggests a crucial role of superoxide in infertility and/or miscarriage in these diseases.

A lot of studies showed the effect of adenomyosis on fertility in patients, who underwent ART. Recent reviews by Vercellini et al. [37] and Younes et al. [38] allowed to shed light on many questions, even though the number of publications analyzed in these reviews is small. In Vercellini review 1865 women were enrolled in the 9 selected studies, and in Younes paper only 15 studies were analyzed.

The prevalence of adenomyosis in the infertility population undergoing IVF/ICSI varies widely, from 6.9% [39] to 34.3 [40]. A clinical pregnancy after IVF/ICSI happens in 40.5% of women with adenomyosis and in 49.8% in those without this disease. The effect of adenomyosis on implantation rate per cycle is still controversial, and different authors have different data, related to that topic [40, 41]. According to Piver's publication [42], JZ thickness could be a predictive factor of repeated implantation failure in women who underwent IVF, suggesting that adenomyosis may impair embryo implantation in IVF cycles. As for the miscarriage rate, we now know that adenomyosis almost doubles this index: 31.9%, compared to 14.1% in women without adenomyosis. There could be also a connection between the miscarriage rate and a live birth rate per cycle. Martínez-Conejero et al. [40] reported 26.8% in the adenomyosis group and of 37.1% in the no adenomyosis group.

Despite the fact that now we have such meta-analysis data, it is still hard to understand the exact influence of the adenomyosis on the fertility, as in some analyzed studies there were groups of patients with both adenomyosis and endometriosis, so it is difficult to identify whether IVF failure and early pregnancy complications were directly related to the presence of endometriosis or the presence of adenomyosis. However, Vercellini and his team concluded that adenomyosis has a negative effect on the outcome of IVF/ICSI, which leads to reduced rates of clinical pregnancy and implantation and an increased risk of early pregnancy loss. To sum up, it seems logical to screen for adenomyosis before starting assisted reproduction procedures [43].

Another publication shows that there is a heightened risk of preterm delivery in patients with adenomyosis. A case–control study of Juang et al. [44] reveals the connection between adenomyosis and preterm birth, and two other studies show poor pregnancy and perinatal outcomes in adenomyosis patients [45, 50].

According to Sandberg's study [46], the prevalence of adenomyosis in women in the time of delivery is quite high (17.8%), but complications during spontaneous pregnancy in such patients are rare. They can include rapid growth in pregnancy [47], spontaneous rupture of an unscarred uterus [48], and delayed postpartum hemorrhage [49]. Also, there is data that women with adenomyosis are at an increased risk of second-trimester miscarriage, small-for-gestational-age, preeclampsia, fetal malpresentation, placental malposition, and postpartum hemorrhage [50]. However, there are no large studies investigating the influence of adenomyosis on perinatal complications, and further accumulation of data is required to reveal this issue. Taking into account that the majority of pregnancies will be uneventful, it may be best that available information should be given to pregnant women in a way that would avoid raising unnecessary anxiety [43].

5.1 Fertily-sparing treatment

Treatment of adenomyosis could be conservative and surgical. Medical treatment for adenomyosis follows the principles for medical treatment of endometriosis, which aim is to reduce the production of endogenic estrogen or induction of endometrial differentiation with progestins. The principles are inhibition of ovulation, abolition of menstruation, and establishment of a stable steroid milieu [51].

Nowadays there are several different options of conservative treatment, mainly against menstruation-related symptoms such as dysmenorrhea and heavy menstrual bleeding. According to Streuli et al. review [52], there are almost no well-conducted randomized controlled trials on the pharmacological treatment of adenomyosis, and the information collected from published studies is insufficient. However, experts' opinion in this review says that the use of levonorgestrel-releasing intrauterine system, oral contraceptive pills, and danazol can improve those symptoms. Also, there are very few reports showing therapeutic effects of these drugs for infertility. Despite the fact that there are many therapeutic options, the majority of them inhibits the ovulation and\or inducts of necrosis, which is unacceptable in infertile patients. So, in this chapter, we will discuss options, which could be applied in such a group of patients.

The use of gonadotropin-releasing hormone agonists (GnRH-a) and its effect on infertility were described in several studies. In two IVF studies [53] in which a long protocol GnRH-a was admitted, there were no lower pregnancy rates in women with adenomyosis. GnRH-a could be admitted in women with moderate to severe symptomatic adenomyosis, especially in women with failed implantation of embryos of high quality. The weak point of these studies is that both of them were retrospective, and other factors may also have contributed. In patients with adenomyosis who plan to have frozen embryo transfer, one study [54] showed that 2-month GnRH analog pretreatment improved rates of implantation, clinical pregnancy, and ongoing pregnancy.

There is also data that the treatment of an intrauterine device containing danazol resulted in the successful conception of infertile patients [55].

5.2 Surgical treatment

Grimbizis reviewed studies on uterus-sparing surgical treatment options for adenomyosis and concluded that this kind of treatment is feasible and efficient [56].

There are several options nowadays: adenomyomectomy for diffuse or focal adenomyosis, cytoreductive surgery (partial adenomyomectomy), or a variety of non-excisional techniques (endometrial ablation, high-intensity focused ultrasound (HIFU) and uterine artery embolization (UAE)). Non-excisional techniques result in tissue necrosis, which is unacceptable in patients who desires pregnancy.

In patients with adenomyosis who desires pregnancy, surgery should only be chosen if the medical treatment is no effect. In patients with the localized process (adenomyoma) it is possible to perform an adenomyomectomy and remove all pathologic tissue. Nowadays it is the most popular surgical technique, performed through the laparoscopic or open approach. Laparoscopic surgery (adenomyosis resection) might be proper for women younger than 40 years old with focal adenomyosis who failed infertility treatments including assisted reproductive technology [57]. Several kinds of incisions are proposed for such procedure—transverse, longitudinal, wedge-shaped, and transverse H-shaped incisions [58], which could be chosen according to the size and location of the lesion. As well as for the incisions, for suturing wounds, there are several different techniques, including double- and triple-flap methods [59, 60].

In **Figure 3** you can see the different types of complete adenomyomectomy.

In patients with the diffuse process, cytoreductive surgery is performed. The main aim of the uterine preservation surgery is quite challenging—to remove the adenomyotic tissue as much as possible and to preserve the functional myometrium to save a functional uterus. In cases of diffuse process, it could be quite difficult to find the right plane and the border between those two layers in the adenomyotic uterus, as the pathologic tissue invades the myometrium. On one side of the scale, there is a radical treatment and on the other a functional uterus.

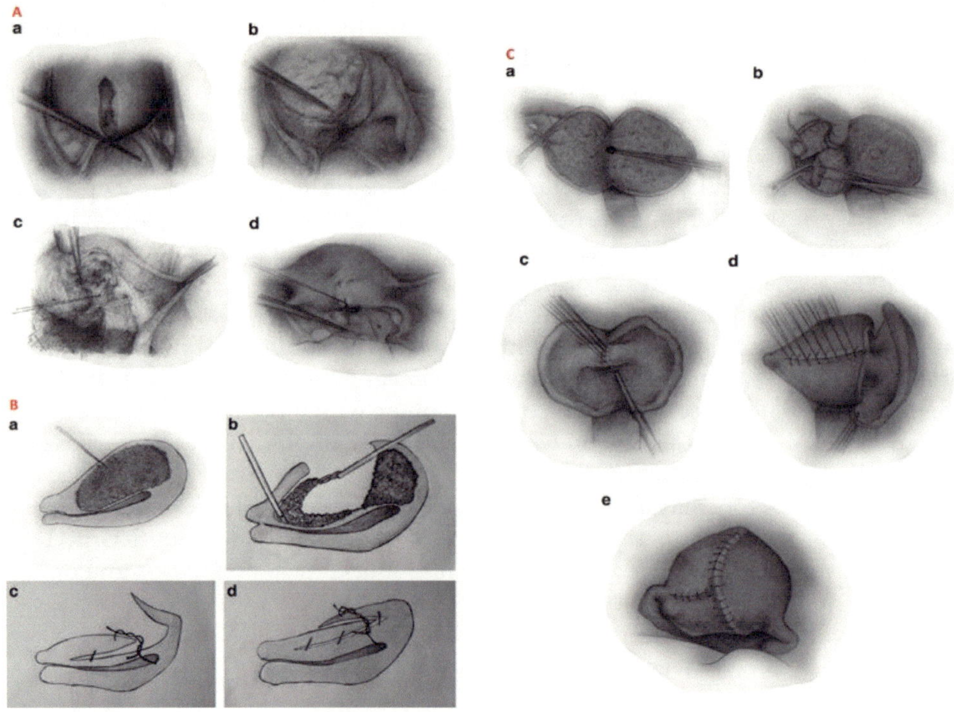

Figure 3.
Different complete adenomyomectomy techniques. (A) Classic technique, (B) classic technique with overlapping flaps, and (C) triple-flap technique [56].

In the recent review of fertility-sparing treatment for adenomyosis by Rocha et al. [61], there is also an analysis of combined medical and surgical treatment. The overall pooled clinical pregnancy rate after surgical resection of adenomyosis was 38.8%, ranging from 12.5 to 61.5%. The pooled miscarriage rate was 17.9% and pooled live birth rate 30.4%. As for spontaneous pregnancies, the overall clinical pregnancy rate was very low (18.2%). However, when using GnRH-a for 24 weeks after surgery [62, 63], the pooled spontaneous pregnancy rate was higher than not using adjuvant GnRH-a. There was no significant difference between pooled results with or without GnRH-a after adenomyomectomy for pregnancy rate, live birth rate, IVF pregnancy rate, or miscarriage rate. Two studies examined the effect of combined treatment with the use of adenomyomectomy and GnRH-a versus GnRH-a treatment alone [62, 64]. Even though the number of patients in the studies was small, it appears that surgery is associated with increased pregnancy rate. To sum up, adenomyomectomy alone has low spontaneous pregnancy rates and should be followed by ART or medical therapy with GnRH-a. Assisted reproductive technologies have good pregnancy rates in women with adenomyosis, and data suggest that long stimulation protocol is superior to short protocol. Most authors agree that there is currently no convincing evidence of the superiority of one of the methods of treatment over another and further prospective studies are needed to elucidate the usefulness of adenomyosis cytoreductive surgery as a fertility treatment. Also at the moment, literature data on such complications like uterine rupture and placenta accrete after surgery is scarce.

There is also a place for treatment adenomyosis with hysteroscopic techniques [65]. This method could be performed in patients with adenomyotic cysts, and crypts are suggested before treatment for fertility [66]. However, this procedure and its effect on adenomyosis are described only in case reports.

Dueholm et al. [51] in the recent review proposed an algorithm of how the patient with adenomyosis should be treated in infertility clinic. This algorithm is presented in **Figure 4**. However, authors make a conclusion that this algorithm is based on limited evidence and further randomized controlled trials are necessary to define the best strategy for patients with adenomyosis who want to conceive.

In the twenty-first century, new technologies come for patients suffering from uterine infertility, and without the option of surrogate motherhood, uterine

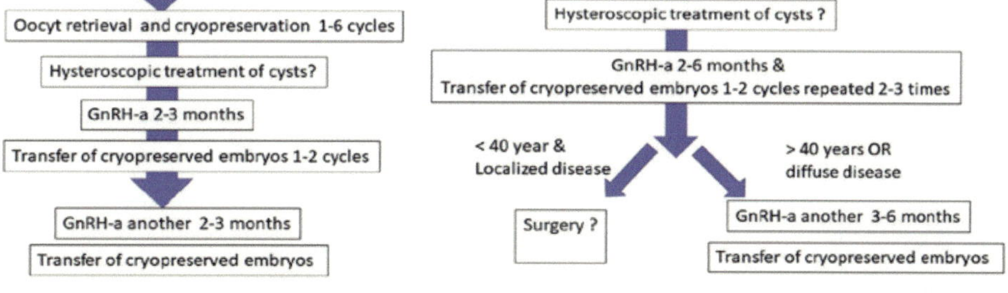

Figure 4.
Treatment algorithm for the patient with adenomyosis in an infertility clinic [51].

transplantation could be the only way to parenthood. Since the report in 2014 of a successful pregnancy [67] in the transplanted uterus, research interest in this field has been steadily growing with an increasing number of surgical teams training on the technique. Thirty-seven transplantations have already been realized worldwide setting the stage for a complex new research area in gynecological surgery, which needs to address technical, ethical, social, and economic issues [68]. These new technologies in the nearest future could also give a chance to become a mother for patients with uterine infertility caused by adenomyosis, resistant to other types of treatment.

6. Summary

In spite of huge achievements both in reproductive surgery and assisted reproductive technologies, endometriosis as a disease is very actual today. It is known that the number of ART centers has been increased recently, the majority of which do not have facilities to perform surgery. This fact seems quite controversial. It resulted in the situation when the importance of reproductive surgery is neglected. Most of the studies are originally oriented to a recognition of ART as a major method of infertility treatment. We think this practice leads to the loss of reproductive surgery quality and professional degradation. Spontaneous pregnancy rate occurs in 30–70% infertile patients after an adequate operation performed just in time. That means one- or two-thirds of patients with endometriosis-associated infertility do not need ART at all. However, surgery is not the only possible kind of infertility treatment. It is important to diminish the number of the second (third, fourth, etc.) surgery. The reproductologist should be involved in the treatment and ART could be recommended promptly. The best option is to find a balance between surgery and ART, which could be reached through the organization of the multidisciplinary team, "brother in arms" professional connections between the surgeon and the reproductologist. Only working together with a constant search of the best solution on how to reach the pregnancy and informing the infertile patient about all ways of the treatment could lead to success.

Conflict of interest

The authors declare no conflict of interest.

Author details

Popov Alexander*, Koval Alexey, Fedorov Anton, Tyurina Svetlana, Fedotova Irina and Khabibullakh Tamana
Moscow Regional Research Institute of Obstetrics and Gynecology, Moscow, Russia

*Address all correspondence to: gyn_endoscopy@mail.ru

References

[1] Chapron C, Lang J, Leng J, Zhou Y, Zhang X, Xue M, et al. Factors and regional differences associated with endometriosis: A multi-country, case-control study. Advances in Therapy. 2016;**33**(8):1385-1407

[2] Nnoaham K, Hummelshoj L, Webster P, d'Hooghe T, de Cicco Nardone F, de Cicco Nardone C, et al. Impact of endometriosis on quality of life and work productivity: A multicenter study across ten countries. Fertility and Sterility. 2011;**96**(2):366-373.e8

[3] Dunselman G, Vermeulen N, Becker C, Calhaz-Jorge C, D'Hooghe T, De Bie B, et al. ESHRE guideline: Management of women with endometriosis. Human Reproduction. 2014;**29**(3):400-412

[4] Vercellini P, Trespidi L, De Giorgi O, Cortesi I, Parazzini F, Crosignani P. Endometriosis and pelvic pain: Relation to disease stage and localization. Presented at the 50th Annual Meeting of The American Fertility Society, San Antonio, Texas, November 5-10, 1994. Fertility and Sterility. 1996;**65**(2):299-304

[5] Vercellini P, Fedele L, Aimi G, De Giorgi O, Consonni D, Crosignani P. Reproductive performance, pain recurrence and disease relapse after conservative surgical treatment for endometriosis: The predictive value of the current classification system. Human Reproduction. 2006;**21**(10):2679-2685

[6] Endometriosis and infertility: A committee opinion. Fertility and Sterility. 2012;**98**(3):591-598

[7] Zeng C, Xu J, Zhou Y, Zhou Y, Zhu S, Xue Q. Reproductive performance after surgery for endometriosis: Predictive value of the Revised American Fertility Society Classification and the Endometriosis Fertility Index. Gynecologic and Obstetric Investigation. 2014;**77**(3):180-185

[8] Ploteau S, Merlot B, Roman H, Canis M, Collinet P, Fritel X. Endométriose minime à légère: Résultats du traitement chirurgical sur la douleur et l'infertilité et modalités techniques. Quelles stratégies thérapeutiques? RPC Endométriose CNGOF-HAS. Gynécologie Obstétrique Fertilité & Sénologie. 2018;**46**(3):273-277

[9] de Ziegler D, Borghese B, Chapron C. Endometriosis and infertility: Pathophysiology and management. The Lancet. 2010;**376**(9742):730-738

[10] Kyama CM, Overbergh L, Mihalyi A, et al. Endometrial and peritoneal expression of aromatase, cytokines, and adhesion factors in women with endometriosis. Fertility and Sterility. 2008;**89**:301-310

[11] Koninckx P, Martin D. Deep endometriosis: A consequence of infiltration or retraction or possibly adenomyosis externa? International Journal of Gynecology & Obstetrics. 1993;**42**(1):89-90

[12] Chapron C, Fauconnier A, Vieira M, Barakat H, Dousset B, Pansini V, et al. Anatomical distribution of deeply infiltrating endometriosis: Surgical implications and proposition for a classification. Human Reproduction. 2003;**18**:157-161

[13] Anaf V, El Nakadi I, Simon P, Van de Stadt J, Fayt I, Simonart T, et al. Preferential infiltration of large bowel endometriosis along the nerves of the colon. Human Reproduction. 2004;**19**:996-1002

[14] Daraï E, Cohen J, Ballester M. Colorectal endometriosis and fertility.

European Journal of Obstetrics & Gynecology and Reproductive Biology. 2017;**209**:86-94

[15] Iversen M, Seyer-Hansen M, Forman A. Does surgery for deep infiltrating bowel endometriosis improve fertility? A systematic review. Acta Obstetricia et Gynecologica Scandinavica. 2017;**96**(6):688-693

[16] Donnez J, Squifflet J. Complications, pregnancy and recurrence in a prospective series of 500 patients operated on by the shaving technique for deep rectovaginal endometriotic nodules. Human Reproduction. 2010;**25**(8):1949-1958

[17] Abrao MS, Petraglia F, Falcone T, Keckstein J, Osuga Y, Chapron C. Deep endometriosis infiltrating the recto-sigmoid: Critical factors to consider before management. Human Reproduction Update. 2015;**21**(3):329-339

[18] Malzoni M, Di Giovanni A, Exacoustos C, Lannino G, Capece R, Perone C, et al. Laparoscopic assisted bowel resection for deep infiltrating endometriosis feasibility and safety: A retrospective cohort study with description of technique. The Journal of Minimally Invasive Gynecology. 2016;**23**(4):512-525. DOI: 10.1016/j.jmig.2015.09.024

[19] Exacoustos C, Lauriola I, Lazzeri L, De Felice G, Zupi E. Complications during pregnancy and delivery in women with untreated rectovaginal deep infiltrating endometriosis. Fertility and Sterility. 2016;**106**(5):1129-1135.e1. DOI: 10.1016/j.fertnstert.2016.06.024

[20] Leyland N, Casper R, Laberge P, Singh S, Allen L, Arendas K, et al. Endometriosis: Diagnosis and management. Journal of Endometriosis. 2010;**2**(3):107-134

[21] Tsoumpou I, Kyrgiou M, Gelbaya TA, Nardo LG. The effect of surgical treatment for endometrioma on in vitro fertilization outcomes: A systematic review and meta-analysis. Fertility and Sterility. 2009;**92**(1):75-87

[22] García-Tejedor A, Castellarnau M, Ponce J, Fernández M, Burdio F. Ethanol sclerotherapy of ovarian endometrioma: A safe and effective minimal invasive procedure. Preliminary results. European Journal of Obstetrics & Gynecology and Reproductive Biology. 2015;**187**:25-29

[23] Somigliana E, Benaglia L, Paffoni A, Busnelli A, Vigano P, Vercellini P. Risks of conservative management in women with ovarian endometriomas undergoing IVF. Human Reproduction Update. 2015;**21**(4):486-499

[24] Hricak H, Alpers C, Crooks LE, Sheldon PE. Magnetic resonance imaging of the female pelvis: Initial experience. American Journal of Roentgenology. 1983;**141**:1119-1128

[25] Luciano DE, Exacoustos C, Albrecht L, Lamonica R, Proffer A, Zupi E, et al. Three-dimensional ultrasound in diagnosis of adenomyosis: Histologic correlation with ultrasound targeted biopsies of the uterus. Journal of Minimally Invasive Gynecology. 2013;**20**:803-810

[26] Ferenczy A. Pathophysiology of adenomyosis. Human Reproduction Update. 1998;**4**(4):312-322

[27] Fauconnier A, Chapron C. Endometriosis and pelvic pain: Epidemiological evidence of the relationship and implications. Human Reproduction Update. 2005;**11**:595-606

[28] Gupta S, Goldberg JM, Aziz N, Goldberg E, Krajcir N, Agarwal A. Pathogenic mechanisms in endometriosis-associated infertility. Fertility and Sterility. 2008;**90**:247-257

[29] Huang FJ, Kung FT, Chang SY, Hsu TY. Effects of short-course buserelin

therapy on adenomyosis: A report of two cases. Journal of Reproductive Medicine for the Obstetrician and Gynecologist. 1999;**44**(8):741-744

[30] Campo S, Campo V, Benagiano G. Adenomyosis and infertility. Reproductive Biomedicine Online. 2012;**24**:35-46

[31] Kunz G, Beil D, Huppert P, Noe M, Kissler S, Leyendecker G. Adenomyosis in endometriosis—Prevalence and impact on fertility. Evidence from magnetic resonance imaging. Human Reproduction. 2005;**20**:2309-2316

[32] Kunz G, Herbertz M, Beil D, Huppert G, Leyendecker G. Adenomyosis as a disorder of the early and late human reproductive period. Reproductive Biomedicine Online. 2007;**15**:681-685

[33] Birnholz JC. Ultrasonic visualization of endometrial movements. Fertility and Sterility. 1984;**41**:157-158

[34] Benagiano G, Brosens I. The endometrium in adenomyosis. Women's Health. 2012;**8**:301-312

[35] Igarashi S, Sato N, Tanaka H, Tanaka T. Involvement of catalase in the endometrium of patients with endometriosis and adenomyosis. Fertility and Sterility. 2002;**78**:804-809

[36] Ota H, Igarashi S, Hatazawa M, Tanaka T. Immunohistochemical assessment of superoxide dismutase expression in the endometrium in endometriosis and adenomyosis. Fertility and Sterility. 1999;**72**:129-134

[37] Vercellini P, Consonni D, Dridi D, Bracco B, Frattaruolo M, Somigliana E. Uterine adenomyosis and in vitro fertilization outcome: A systematic review and meta-analysis. Human Reproduction. 2014;**29**(5):964-977

[38] Younes G, Tulandi T. Effects of adenomyosis on in vitro fertilization treatment outcomes: A meta-analysis. Fertility and Sterility. 2017;**108**(3): 483-490.e3

[39] Salim R, Riris S, Saab W, Abramov B, Khadum I, Serhal P. Adenomyosis reduces pregnancy rates in infertile women undergoing IVF. Reproductive Biomedicine Online. 2012;**25**:273-277

[40] Martínez-Conejero JA, Morgan M, Montesinos M, Fortuño S, Meseguer M, Simón C, et al. Adenomyosis does not affect implantation, but is associated with miscarriage in patients undergoing oocyte donation. Fertility and Sterility. 2011;**96**:943-950

[41] Mijatovic V, Florijn E, Halim N, Schats R, Hompes P. Adenomyosis has no adverse effects on IVF/ICSI outcomes in women with endometriosis treated with long-term pituitary down-regulation before IVF/ICSI. European Journal of Obstetrics & Gynecology and Reproductive Biology. 2010;**151**:62-65

[42] Piver P. Uterine factors limiting ART coverage. Journal de Gynécologie Obstétrique et Biologie de la Reproduction. 2005;**34**(7 Pt 2):5S30-5S33

[43] Benagiano G, Brosens I, Habiba M. Adenomyosis: A life-cycle approach. Reproductive Bio Medicine Online. 2015;**30**(3):220-232

[44] Juang CM, Chou P, Yen MS, Twu NF, Horng HC, Hsu WL. Adenomyosis and risk of preterm delivery. BJOG: An International Journal of Obstetrics and Gynaecology. 2007;**114**(2):165-169

[45] Mochimaru A, Aoki S, Oba MS, Kurasawa K, Takahashi T, Hirahara F. Adverse pregnancy outcomes associated with adenomyosis with uterine enlargement. The Journal of Obstetrics and Gynaecology Research. 2015;**41**(4): 529-533

[46] Sandberg EC, Cohn F. Adenomyosis in the gravid uterus at term. American

Journal of Obstetrics and Gynecology. 1962;**84**:1457-1465

[47] Kim SH, Kim JK, Chae HD, Kim CH, Kang BM. Rapidly growing adenomyosis during the first trimester: Magnetic resonance images. Fertility and Sterility. 2006;**85**:1057-1058

[48] Nikolaou M, Kourea HP, Antonopoulos K, Geronatsiou K, Adonakis G, Decavalas G. Spontaneous uterine rupture in a primigravid woman in the early third trimester attributed to adenomyosis: A case report and review of the literature. The Journal of Obstetrics and Gynaecology Research. 2013;**39**:727-732

[49] Wang P-H, Pang Y-P, Chao H-T, Lai C-R, Juang C-M, Yuan C-C, et al. Delayed postpartum hemorrhage in adenomyosis: A case report. Chinese Medical Journal (Taipei). 1998;**61**:492-495

[50] Hashimoto A, Iriyama T, Sayama S, Nakayama T, Komatsu A, Miyauchi A, et al. Adenomyosis and adverse perinatal outcomes: Increased risk of second trimester miscarriage, preeclampsia, and placental malposition. The Journal of Maternal-Fetal & Neonatal Medicine. 2018;**31**:1-6

[51] Dueholm M. Minimally invasive treatment of adenomyosis. Best Practice & Research Clinical Obstetrics & Gynaecology. 2018;**51**:119-137

[52] Streuli I, Dubuisson J, Santulli P, de Ziegler D, Batteux F, Chapron C. An update on the pharmacological management of adenomyosis. Expert Opinion on Pharmacotherapy. 2014;**15**(16):2347-2360

[53] Costello MF, Lindsay K, McNally G. The effect of adenomyosis on in vitro fertilisation and intra-cytoplasmic sperm injection treatment outcome. European Journal of Obstetrics & Gynecology and Reproductive Biology. 2011;**158**(2):229-234

[54] Niu Z, Chen Q, Sun Y, Feng Y. Long-term pituitary downregulation before frozen embryo transfer could improve pregnancy outcomes in women with adenomyosis. Gynecological Endocrinology. 2013;**29**(12):1026-1030

[55] Igarashi M, Abe Y, Fukuda M, Ando A, Miyasaka M, Yoshida M, et al. Novel conservative medical therapy for uterine adenomyosis with a danazol-loaded intrauterine device. Fertility and Sterility. 2000;**74**(2):412-413

[56] Grimbizis GF, Mikos T, Tarlatzis B. Uterus-sparing operative treatment for adenomyosis. Fertility and Sterility. 2014;**101**:472e87

[57] Wang CJ, Yuen LT, Chang SD, Lee CL, Soong YK. Use of laparoscopic cytoreductive surgery to treat infertile women with localized adenomyosis. Fertility and Sterility. 2006;**86**(2):462.e5-e8

[58] Fujishita A, Masuzaki H, Khan KN, Kitajima M, Ishimaru T. Modified reduction surgery for adenomyosis. A preliminary report of the transverse H incision technique. Gynecologic and Obstetric Investigation. 2004;**57**(3):132-138

[59] Huang X, Huang Q, Chen S, Zhang J, Lin K, Zhang X. Efficacy of laparoscopic adenomyomectomy using double-flap method for diffuse uterine adenomyosis. BMC Women's Health. 2015;**15**:24

[60] Osada H, Silber S, Kakinuma T, Nagaishi M, Kato K, Kato O. Surgical procedure to conserve the uterus for future pregnancy in patients suffering from massive adenomyosis. Reproductive Biomedicine Online. 2011;**22**(1):94-99

[61] Rocha T, Andres M, Borrelli G, Abrão M. Fertility-sparing treatment of adenomyosis in patients with infertility: A systematic review of

current options. Reproductive Sciences. 2018;**25**(4):480-486

[62] Al Jama FE. Management of adenomyosis in subfertile women and pregnancy outcome. Oman Medical Journal. 2011;**26**(3):178-181

[63] Huang BS, Seow KM, Tsui KH, Huang CY, Lu YF, Wang PH. Fertility outcome of infertile women with adenomyosis treated with the combination of a conservative microsurgical technique and GnRH agonist: long-term follow-up in a series of nine patients. Taiwanese Journal of Obstetrics and Gynecology. 2012;**51**(2):212-216

[64] Wang PH, Liu WM, Fuh JL, Cheng MH, Chao HT. Comparison of surgery alone and combined surgical-medical treatment in the management of symptomatic uterine adenomyoma. Fertility and Sterility. 2009;**92**(3):876-885

[65] Di Spiezio Sardo A, Calagna G, Santangelo F, Zizolfi B, Tanos V, Perino A, et al. The role of hysteroscopy in the diagnosis and treatment of adenomyosis. BioMed Research International. 2017;**2017**:2518396

[66] Gordts S, Campo R, Brosens I. Hysteroscopic diagnosis and excision of myometrial cystic adenomyosis. Gynecological Surgery. 2014;**11**:273e8

[67] Brännström M, Johannesson L, Bokström H, et al. Livebirth after uterus transplantation. Lancet. 2015;**385**(9968):607-616

[68] Favre-Inhofer A, Rafii A, Carbonnel M, Revaux A, Ayoubi J. Uterine transplantation: Review in human research. Journal of Gynecology Obstetrics and Human Reproduction. 2018;**47**(6):213-221

Section 5

Endometriosis Treatment

Chapter 7

Interventional Treatment of Endometriosis

Yang Xiaomin, Han Jun, Feng Pin and Yang Xiaojun

Abstract

Patients with endometriosis and adenomyosis naturally improve after menopause. Therefore, some patients only need to relieve symptoms, especially those near menopause, and they prefer to be treated by conservative methods. We summarized several minimally invasive interventional methods: uterine artery intervention (Uterine artery embolization, UAE), nerve intervention (upper and lower abdominal plexus block, SHPB), ultrasound intervention (puncture sclerotherapy; high intensity focused ultrasound treatment).

Keywords: superior hypogastric plexus block, uterine artery embolization, ultrasound interventional

1. Introduction

Adenomyosis and endometriosis are common gynecological diseases. Most of the patients are primipara aged 35–50 years old. About half of the patients have hysteromyoma at the same time. Clinical manifestations are dysmenorrhea, menstrual disorders, and enlargement of the uterine body. Secondary dysmenorrhea and Menorrhagia are the most typical symptoms of this disease [1].

The main symptom of endometriosis is progressive secondary dysmenorrhea which severely affects patient's quality of life. Menorrhagia caused by adenomyosis may lead to severe anemia in some patients. The treatment is often personalized and optimized according to disease severity and patient age. At present, there are several non-surgical conservative treatments for secondary dysmenorrhea and menorrhagia.

2. Minimally invasive interventional therapies

2.1 Uterine artery embolization (UAE)

UAE is the treatment of symptomatic uterine fibroids by embolizing the vascular network of the lesion after reaching the uterine artery through the intervention, which blocks the blood supply of the lesion [2]. It was first reported in 1995 by Ravina et al. This technique has the characteristics of uterus preservation, easy operation, rapid postoperative recovery, and less postoperative complications and has become one of the effective minimally invasive alternatives in the treatment of symptomatic uterine adenomyosis. The American College of Obstetricians and Gynecologists (ACOG) has recommended UAE as a safe and effective treatment option for patients with uterine fibroids who wish to preserve the uterus (level A evidence) [3]. Therefore, UAE has been widely used in the treatment of uterine leiomyoma, and then UAE has achieved significant effect in the treatment of pain and anemia symptoms of adenomyosis, but there is controversy in the use of adenomyosis, which may recur after a period of time due to symptoms [4]. In recent years, more and more literatures show that UAE is effective in the treatment of adenomyosis, especially in the short term [5–7]. UAE treatment alleviated the symptoms of adenomyosis and made most adenomyosis patients retain the uterus [8].

2.1.1 Rationale for UAE in uterine adenomyosis

Adenomyosis is a diffuse or local proliferation of surrounding smooth muscle and fibrous connective tissue caused by glandular and stromal invasion of the basal layer of the endometrium, and the ectopic endometrium is in the proliferative phase due to its origin from the basal layer of the endometrium. The above lesions have a relatively rich network of new blood vessels and poor tolerance to ischemia and hypoxia, but the normal uterine tissue has a rich vascular traffic network, and the normal uterus has a strong tolerance to ischemia and hypoxia. Embolization of the vascular network of the lesion through the uterine artery blocks the blood supply of the lesion (after), resulting in ischemic necrosis of the lesion, followed by dissolution and absorption, and finally the lesion shrinks or even disappears, while the reduction of the lesion reduces the uterine volume and uterine cavity area, which can effectively reduce the menstrual volume, so as to achieve the purpose of relieving symptoms.

2.1.2 Indications and contraindications of UAE

2.1.2.1 Indications

(1) Patients are willing to undergo UAE treatment and understand the relevant possible complications. (2) Symptomatic adenomyosis without fertility requirements, including dysmenorrhea and heavy menstrual bleeding. (3) Patients with uterine adenomyosis who fail non-surgical treatment or refuse surgery or have a history of multiple surgeries and are difficult to treat by reoperation. (4) Patients with pelvic endometriosis (including ovarian endometrioma) at the same time, need to inform UAE is ineffective for the above disease, in patients with full understanding and requirements, the option of UAE treatment of adenomyosis combined with laparoscopic treatment of pelvic endometriosis (including ovarian endometrioma). (5) Patients with symptomatic uterine adenomyosis who have fertility requirements should use UAE with caution. In terms of indications, we have repeatedly stressed that UAE should be carefully selected for patients with adenomyosis who have fertility requirements. The reason is that the medium- and long-term effects of UAE on endometrial microcirculation or intrauterine environment is still uncertain. UAE needs to be performed under X-ray. The skill level of the operator and the vascular condition of the patient are linear, which will affect the amount of radiation received by the patient, and the effect of radiation on the fertility rate is also uncertain. This kind of research is rare, because it involves ethical review and cannot be passed.

2.1.2.2 Contraindications

(1) Pregnant women; (2) combined with genitourinary system infection; (3) known or suspected gynecological malignant tumors coexist; (4) general contraindications of interventional embolization therapy, such as contrast agent allergy,

puncture site skin infection, renal insufficiency, or severe immunosuppression of the body; and (5) patients with uterine fibroids or adenomyosis whose lesions are mainly supplied by the ovarian artery [9].

2.1.3 Preoperative evaluation of UAE

2.1.3.1 History and evaluation

These include detailed gynecological history, such as menstrual history, previous pregnancy, fertility plan, gynecological disease, and previous pelvic surgery, medical history to identify various comorbidities, and previous use of anticoagulants. Adequate informed consent is required, and informed consent for surgical procedures is signed to understand the advantages and disadvantages of treatment, expected effects, and potential complications.

2.1.3.2 Evaluation of dysmenorrhea

A comprehensive assessment of the degree of recent and long-term dysmenorrhea in patients with adenomyosis was performed using the visual analog scale (VAS) for pain and the chronic pain rating scale. The clinical evaluation standard of dysmenorrhea symptoms: the degree of dysmenorrhea was evaluated by chronic pain rating scale before and after operation. We used VAS to evaluate the degree of dysmenorrhea at each follow-up time point, and VAS weighted calculation method to evaluate the efficacy of UAE in the treatment of dysmenorrhea in adenomyosis. Effective: the postoperative dysmenorrhea disappeared or the postoperative dysmenorrhea symptoms existed, but the score of chronic pain rating scale decreased by two or more levels, (1) cured: (preoperative VAS score – postoperative VAS score)/preoperative VAS score × 100% ≥ 75%; (2) effective: (preoperative VAS score – postoperative VAS score)/preoperative VAS score × 100% ≥ 50% and < 75%; (3) effective: (preoperative VAS score – postoperative VAS score)/preoperative VAS score × 100% ≥ 25% and < 50%. No effect: the symptoms of dysmenorrhea after operation exist, the score of chronic pain rating scale is only reduced by one grade, or the dysmenorrhea is not relieved or even continues to increase, or (preoperative VAS score – postoperative VAS score)/preoperative VAS score × 100% < 25%.

2.1.3.3 Clinical evaluation criteria for menstrual volume

Menorrhagia was defined as menstrual flow >80 ml per menstrual cycle (more than 20 sanitary napkins were used); oligomenorrhea was defined as menstrual flow <5 ml per menstrual cycle (less than 1 sanitary napkin was used). Clinical evaluation standard of menstrual volume: subjective symptoms of patients. Significant effect: after UAE treatment, menstrual volume decreased significantly. Effective: after UAE treatment, menstrual volume decreased. No effect: after UAE treatment, the menstrual volume was not significantly reduced.

2.1.3.4 Examination before treatment

In addition to routine preoperative examinations, sex hormone levels were measured to assess ovarian function. Because the influence of uterine artery embolization on ovarian function is uncertain. Blood CA125 levels were measured for follow-up, CA125 was used as a follow-up index because we found that most patients with adenomyosis have different degrees of increase in this index.

The reason is that the serum CA125 antigen of patients with this disease is secreted by ectopic endometrium between muscles, and CA125 molecules on the surface of endometrial cells are released into the blood circulation, which increases the concentration of CA125 antigen in the blood. Several studies [10] also show that serum CA125 assay is of great assistance to the diagnosis of uterine adenomyosis. Blood CA125 levels were measured for follow-up. Venous color Doppler ultrasonography of both lower limbs is particularly important to assess the presence or absence of preoperative thrombosis.

2.1.3.5 Imaging evaluation

MRI examination, ultrasonography, CT, and other assessments, which perform the planning of the surgical approach and reduce the blindness of the procedure, can improve the success rate of surgery. By contrast, most studies recommend MRI as the main preoperative evaluation method.

2.1.4 Operating process of UAE

The patient was placed in supine position. Routine disinfection and draping were performed. After local anesthesia, the right femoral artery was punctured by Seldinger method. The catheter sheath was placed. A 5F Cobra catheter was inserted into the opening of bilateral uterine arteries for DSA. The dosage of contrast medium on each side was 6 ml and the flow rate was 2 ml/s. The uterus was significantly enlarged, the uterine artery was significantly thickened and tortuous, and the staining in the uterus was thickened. If there was uterine fibroids, the angiography showed the presence of "holding ball" abnormal vascular mass. The 3F microcatheter was used to superselect to the distal end of the main uterine artery, avoiding the ovarian artery. The uterine artery was embolized with embolic agent. The DSA was reexamined. The abnormal staining of the uterus disappeared, and the main uterine artery was retained. The operation could be ended.

2.1.4.1 Selection of embolic agent

There are many embolization agents available for UAE. Generally, particle embolization agents are selected. Generally, they can be divided into absorbable and non-absorbable. Absorbable embolization agents are represented by gelatin sponge particles, and non-absorbable embolization agents are represented by polyvinyl alcohol embolization microspheres (embosphere). However, the commonly used embolic agents of other organs, such as steel ring, absolute ethanol, and super-liquid iodized oil, are not recommended for use in UAE. For the selection of embolic agent particle size, "sandwich embolization" should be used for embolization of uterine adenomyosis due to the small inner vascular network. First, particles with a diameter of 100–300 μm are selected for embolization of the inner vascular network, particles with a diameter of 300–500 μm are used for embolization of the outer vascular network, and finally particles with a diameter of 500–700 μm are used for trunk embolization [11]. The effect of arterial embolization is inversely proportional to the embolic agent particle size.

2.1.4.2 Degree of embolism

Embolization is divided into two types: complete embolization and incomplete embolization. Patients with uterine adenomyosis require complete embolization of the inner vascular network of the uterus, and in DSA, imaging findings show complete disappearance of focal staining, visualization of the main trunk of the uterine artery, retention of contrast agent, and no clearance of contrast agent in five cardiac cycles.

2.1.5 Postoperative management of UAE

For hemostasis by compression at the puncture site, the lower limbs were immobilized for 6 h. If a vascular sealer was used, the immobilization time could be shortened. After operation, it is necessary to observe the skin color and skin temperature of lower limbs, ask the dorsalis pedis artery pulse and mark it, and make regular observation to prevent thrombosis. Antibiotics were not routinely applied postoperatively.

2.1.6 Complications of UAE

2.1.6.1 Intraoperative complications

1. Local bleeding or hematoma: bleeding or hematoma at the puncture site is a more common complication, and severe cases can cause large pelvic retroperitoneal hematoma. Hemostasis by compression was given for symptomatic treatment.

2. Arterial spasm: repeated stimulation of blood vessels or long operation time during surgery may cause arterial spasm, cause limb numbness and pain, affect intraoperative operation, and in severe cases, lead to limb ischemic necrosis. Analgesic drugs can be used to relieve pain and intraoperative application of 2% lidocaine 5 ml local intra-arterial injection.

3. Arterial puncture injury: although arterial puncture injury caused by improper operation or traumatic operation is rare during the operation, because the pelvic artery is located in the retroperitoneum, once it occurs, it will be difficult to compress and stop bleeding, which can form retroperitoneal hematoma. Failure to timely detect it will threaten the patient's life and require emergency laparotomy for hemostasis. Therefore, intraoperative manipulation should be gentle, and the direction of the vessel should be identified when resistance is encountered, homeopathic.

2.1.6.2 Postoperative complications

1. Pain: almost all patients experience pain after surgery. At present, it is believed that pain is associated with ischemia of the lesion and uterus after UAE. The degree of pain varies from mild to severe colic. Analgesic methods depend on the severity of pain and preemptive non-steroidal anti-inflammatory drugs, patient-controlled analgesia, oral or parenteral administration of opioids using analgesic pumps are optional. The duration of pain varies and is generally gradually relieved 2 to 5 days after surgery. If the pain is more than 1 week and more severe, we should be alert to the possibility of serious complications such as secondary infection and thrombosis.

2. Post-embolization syndrome: post-embolization syndrome is characterized by pelvic pain, nausea, vomiting, fever, fatigue, myalgia, discomfort, and leukocytosis. Most of them occurred within 24 h after surgery and gradually improved within 7 days. It is a common postoperative complication. Postoperative fever is generally no higher than 38°C, which is postoperative absorption fever, and antibiotic treatment is usually not required.

3. Arterial rupture or arterial dissection: it is a serious complication and requires surgical repair.

4. Misthrombosis of blood vessels: because the anterior trunk of the internal iliac artery not only gives off the uterine artery but also the bladder artery, vaginal artery, and internal pudendal artery, when the iliac artery and the above arteries are misembolized, complications such as labia majora and minora necrosis and local bladder necrosis may occur.

5. Infection: the operation of UAE is a type I incision, and incision infection is rare, mainly necrosis of the lesion after embolization, forming aseptic inflammation. After uterine artery interventional therapy, uterine ischemic focus atrophied and vaginal secretion increased. At that time, the uterus is prone to secondary bacterial infection, and in the worst case, hysterectomy is needed to control sepsis. Intrauterine adhesions can be seen in long-term complications.

6. Allergic reactions or rashes: anti-allergic treatment may be given.

7. Bloody vaginal discharge: usually within 2 weeks, a very small number may also last for months.

8. Oligomenorrhea: after surgery, some patients have partial endometrial necrosis due to uterine artery vascular network embolization, and menstrual volume may be significantly reduced, but hormone examination shows no significant abnormality. If there is no fertility requirement, this part of patients can be observed without treatment.

9. Amenorrhea: it is a long-term complication of UAE and is divided into ovarian amenorrhea and uterine amenorrhea. Ovarian amenorrhea is mainly caused by ovarian ischemia and necrosis due to blocking of blood flow in the arteries supplying the ovary, such as the ovarian branch of the uterine artery or the ovarian artery and amenorrhea due to ovarian failure, requiring long-term oral administration of hormone drugs to maintain the level of hormones in the body. Uterine amenorrhea is caused by endometrial ischemic necrosis and impaired endometrial growth, which does not affect hormone secretion and can be observed, but the patient is unable to have children.

10. Others: other serious complications are rare. The incidence of venous thromboembolic complications is approximately 0.4%. Rare complications such as fatal sepsis, femoral nerve injury, iliac artery embolism, uterine ischemic infarction, labia majora and minora necrosis, local bladder necrosis, vesicouterine fistula, uterine wall injury, and necrosis of both toes or heels due to extravasation of embolic agents associated with the UAE procedure also occur. Readmission was required in 2.4 to 3.5% of patients and unplanned surgery in 1.0 to 2.5% of patients. However, overall mortality from UAE was not increased compared with hysterectomy [9].

2.1.7 Follow-up time and efficacy evaluation after UAE treatment

2.1.7.1 Follow-up time

After UAE treatment, reexamination assessment is required at 1, 3, and 6 months, and once a year thereafter. The contents of follow-up included change of lesion size, menstruation, sex hormone level, change of dysmenorrhea degree, and CA125 level in patients with adenomyosis.

2.1.7.2 Clinical efficacy evaluation

A large number of clinical trial data [11, 12] showed that 97–100% of patients could tolerate and complete the operation, 77–97.4% of patients had improvement of dysmenorrhea symptoms, and amenorrhea happens occasionally. About 20% of patients need operation or second UAE because of unsatisfactory effect or recurrence of symptoms.

2.2 Nerve intervention: The superior hypogastric plexus block

2.2.1 Rationale for SHPB in uterine adenomyosis

The superior hypogastric plexus consists of the lumbar splanchnic nerves (from the L3–L4 sympathetic ganglia) and the abdominal aortic plexus, which distributes its fibers to the anterior sacral promontory of the L5 vertebral body below the iliac bifurcation of the abdominal aorta [13]. The superior and inferior ventral nerve block was derived from the sacral neurotomy 20 years ago. Under the guidance of CT, the puncture needle was placed around the superior and inferior ventral nerve in front of the cone, and anhydrous alcohol or other nerve blockers were used to block the nerve so that local pain cannot be transmitted back to the brain through the nerve, to achieve the purpose of analgesia [14].

2.2.2 Indications and contraindications of SHPB

2.2.2.1 Indications

(i) An ultrasonogram indicated uterine adenomyosis, with a slight increase of the cancer antigen (CA)-125 or (ii) there was a history of relevant endometriosis operation along with the absence of surgical indications for immediate reoperation. Patients who satisfied either criterion were then included if they met all the following additional criteria: (iii) periodic hypogastric pain during menstruation, with a visual analog scale (VAS) score >6 (severe); (iv) age >40 years; (v) absence of menorrhagia and significant pelvic mass; and (vi) absence of dysmenorrhea due to intrauterine devices. Among the patients who satisfied these criteria, we enrolled those who provided written informed consent to undergo an operation.

2.2.2.2 Contraindications

The contraindications were as follows: (i) Nulliparous; (ii) Complications due to other pelvic diseases; (iii) Acute appendicitis, acute pelvic inflammatory disease; (iv) Deep endometriosis; (v) Allergic to alcohol or iohexol.

2.2.3 Operating process of SHPB

The patient was asked to lie on the CT table with a suitable pillow under the abdomen. After confirming the absence of any contraindications to a neural block, an intravenous infusion channel was opened. CT scans are used to confirm the location of the L5 and S1 intervertebral spaces, which are the target regions for puncture. Then, the coronal CT scan is obtained by taking the puncture space as the midline, including the upper, lower and central sections with a thickness of 3 mm. Select the best puncture section from CT images and plan the puncture path. The anterolateral margin of the lumbar 5 was the left margin and the anterior margin of the psoas major was the right margin. After planning the puncture route and bilateral puncture points, the angle and depth of puncture points were measured with CT ruler. According to the

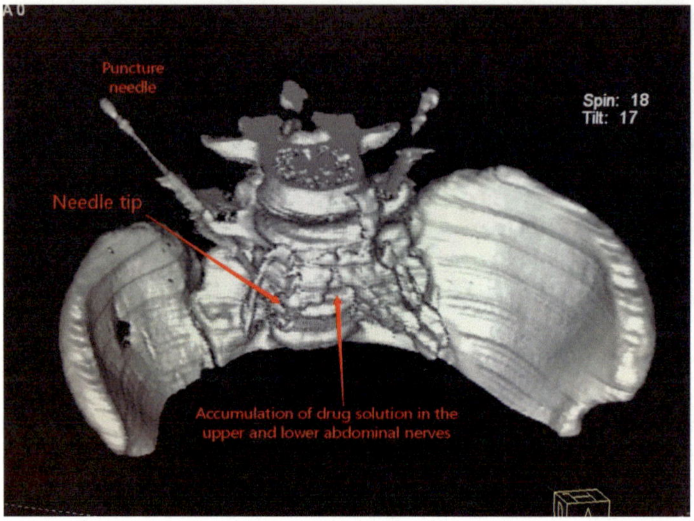

Figure 1.
The upper and lower abdominal nerve block was performed by puncture and injection (Three-dimensional reconstruction by CT).

measurement results, place the puncture needle to the target (**Figure 1**). A solution of 2% lidocaine containing iohexol (a contrast agent) was injected, and its distribution was observed on a CT rescan. An injection site is determined as appropriate if: (i) the lidocaine-iohexol solution is distributed along the anteromedial margin of the psoas major muscle and the anterior vertebral body (**Figure 2**) and (ii) a loss of sensation bilaterally in the lower limbs without dyskinesia is observed after 15 min. With the injection site confirmed, a contrast medium of dehydrated alcohol solution (4 mL) containing 3% iohexol (0.5 mL) is injected bilaterally to achieve a neurolytic block of the superior hypogastric plexus. This is followed by repeated CT, and three-dimensional

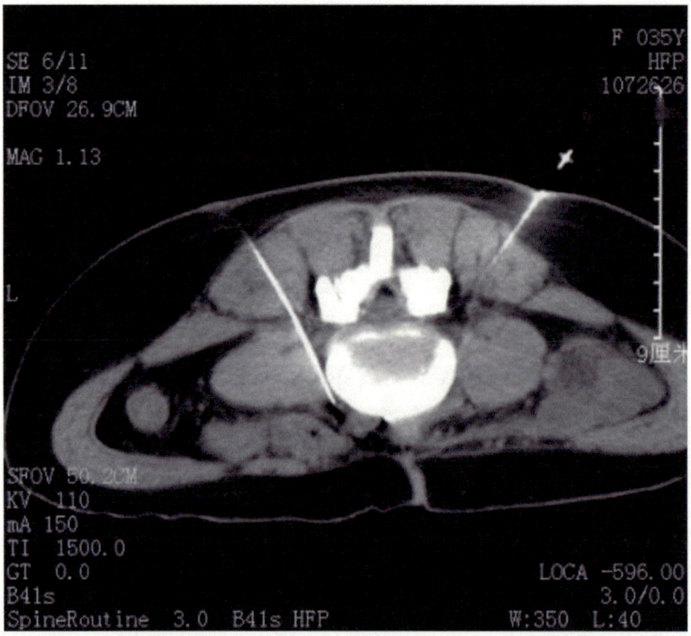

Figure 2.
Upper and lower abdominal nerve block by puncture injection.

reconstruction to observe the distribution of the dehydrated rate, blood pressure. At the same time blood oxygen saturation level is recorded. Any complications are also recorded.

2.2.4 Follow-up time and efficacy evaluation after SHPB treatment

At present, there is no reliable follow-up data of big data, but according to the existing experience, the effective rate is 70%, the duration is 1–3 years, and there is no serious complications related to nerve block. Sacral neurotomy as the predecessor of nerve block treatment appeared 20 years ago, but the technology of nerve block by drugs is still very young. The improvement methods can be as follows: to study the characteristics and efficacy of different nerve blockers, to improve the puncture approach and the position of the blocking point, etc. [15]. SHPB is a new way of treatment. There are no data about future fertility. The upper and lower abdominal nerves are the proximal part of sacral nerves. The same reason is that there are few data at present, which cannot explain the effect of nerve block on fertility, sexual function and urination function.

2.3 Ultrasound interventional therapy for endometriosis

2.3.1 Pelvic endometriosis

Ultrasound-guided puncture sclerotherapy [16], sclerosing agent selection includes anhydrous ethanol, lauryl alcohol, etc. Anhydrous ethanol is less used due to easy to cause low fever, sharp pain, allergies and drunk-like reactions and other adverse reactions poly(lauryl alcohol), the scientific name of polyoxyethylene lauryl alcohol ether, is called polydocanol in Europe. After the injection into the cyst, the protein of the cell will be precipitated quickly, the double molecular layer of the cell wall will be destroyed, the epithelial cells of the cyst wall will be necrotic, the secretion of the fluid of the cell will be inhibited, and the aseptic inflammation will be produced to make the fibrosis of the cyst wall, so as to achieve the purpose of curing the cyst. The drug is widely used. Before the operation, the number and nature of the cyst were confirmed. Under the guidance of real-time ultrasound positioning, the puncture needle entered the center of the cyst, extracted the fluid from the cyst, rinsed the wall of the cyst repeatedly with normal saline, and finally injected with poly(lauryl alcohol) for retention, with a total volume of <50 ml. The results showed that the total effective rate of ultrasound intervention was 93.75%, which had little effect on ovarian reserve function.

2.3.2 Adenomyosis

High intensity (frequency < 1 MHz) focused ultrasound can be used to treat adenomyosis [17]. High intensity focused ultrasound (HIFU) can promote low-frequency and high-energy ultrasound to reach the target tissue through the body surface fat. It makes use of the cavitation, mechanical and thermal effects of ultrasound to induce irreversible damage and degeneration of adenomyosis cells. After the operation, the volume of the lesion was reduced, the symptoms of the patients were relieved, and the treatment process was safe.

3. Conclusions

The symptoms of endometriosis and adenomyosis are different from each other; so, individualized treatment according to different needs of patients is of great significance.

This chapter provides three kinds of conservative treatment methods commonly used in recent years for readers' reference. These three methods either reduce menstrual volume or relieve dysmenorrhea, so that patients avoid surgery; the effect is positive.

Acknowledgements

First and foremost, I would like to show my deepest gratitude to my supervisor, Dr. Yang Xiaojun, a respectable, responsible, and resourceful scholar, who has provided me with valuable guidance in every stage of the writing of this thesis.

I would also like to thank Dr. Huang Bing for his work and research in the treatment of endometriosis with nerve block. Neuromodulation therapy is a new subject. Dr. Huang and his team are studying the use of neuromodulation to treat various refractory diseases in various systems.

Thanks to the first hospital of Jiaxing City, Zhejiang Province, China. They have given some support to complete this chapter. It has contributed to the promotion of conservative treatment of endometriosis.

Conflict of interest

The authors declare no conflict of interest.

Nomenclature

UAE	uterine artery embolization
SHPB	nerve intervention: the superior hypogastric plexus block

Author details

Yang Xiaomin[1], Han Jun[2], Feng Pin[2] and Yang Xiaojun[3]*

1 Jiaxing Hospital of Traditional Chinese Medicine, Zhejiang Chinese Medical University Affiliated Jiaxing TCM Hospital, Jiaxing University Affiliated TCM Hospital, Jiaxing, Zhejiang, China

2 The First Hospital of Jiaxing, Affiliated Hosptial of Jiaxing University, Jiaxing, Zhejiang, China

3 The First Affiliated Hospital of Soochow University, Suzhou, Jiangsu, China

*Address all correspondence to: 12203681@qq.com

References

[1] Zondervan KT et al. Endometriosis. Nature Reviews. Disease Primers. 2018;**4**(1):9

[2] Reidy JF. Uterine artery embolization. Journal of Radiology Nursing. 2008;**27**(2):82-83

[3] ACOG practice bulletin. Alternatives to hysterectomy in themanagement of leiomyomas. Obstetrics and Gynecology. 2008;**112**(2Pt 1):387-400. DOI: 10.1097/AOG.0b013e318183fbab

[4] Bratby MJ, Walker WJ. Uterine artery embolisation for symptomatic adenomyosis—Mid-term results. European Journal of Radiology. 2009;**70**:128-132

[5] Levgur M. Therapeutic options for adenomyosis: A review. Archives of Gynecology and Obstetrics. 2007;**276**:1-15

[6] Jha RC, Takahama J, Imaoka I, et al. Adenomyosis: MRI of the uterus treated with uterine artery embolization. American Journal of Roentgenology. 2003;**181**:851-856

[7] Lohle PN, De Vries J, Klazen CA, Boekkooi PF, Vervest HA, Smeets AJ, et al. Uterine artery embolization for symptomatic adenomyosis with or without uterine leiomyomas with the use of calibrated tris-acryl gelatin microspheres: Midterm clinical and MR imaging follow-up. Journal of Vascular and Interventional Radiology. 2007;**18**:835-841

[8] Smeets AJ, Nijenhuis RJ, Boekkooi PF, et al. Long-term follow-up of uterine artery embolization for symptomatic adenomyosis. Cardiovascular and Interventional Radiology. 2012;**35**:815-819

[9] Bulman JC, Ascher SM, Spies JB. Current concepts in uterine fibroid embolization. Radiographics. 2012;**32**(6):1735-1750. DOI: 10.1148/rg.326125514

[10] Kil K, Chung J-E, Pak HJ, et al. Usefulness of CA125 in the differential diagnosis of uterine adenomyosis and myoma. European Journal of Obstetrics, Gynecology, and Reproductive Biology. 2015;**185**:131-135

[11] Wang S, Xiaomei M, Dong Y. The evaluation of uterine artery embolization as a nonsurgical treatment option for adenomyosis. International Journal of Gynaecology and Obstetrics. 2016;**133**:202-205

[12] Shu S, Tsuyoshi H, Megumi T, et al. Unique learning system for uterine artery embolization for symptomatic myoma and adenomyosis for obstetrician-gynecologists in cooperation with interventional radiologists: Evaluation of UAE from the point of view of gynecologists who perform UAE. Journal of Minimally Invasive Gynecology. 2018;**25**:84-92

[13] Worthington-Kirsch R, Spies JB, Myers ER, et al. The fibroid registry for outcomes data (FIBROID) for uterine embolization: Short-term outcomes. Obstetrics and Gynecology. 2005;**106**(1):52-59. DOI: 10.1097/01.AOG.0000165828.68787.a9

[14] Yang X, You J, Tao S, et al. Computed tomography-guided superior hypogastric plexus block for secondary dysmenorrhea in perimenopausal women. Medical Science Monitor: International Medical Journal of Experimental and Clinical Research. 2018;**24**:5132-5138

[15] Cranney R, Condous G, Reid S. An update on the diagnosis, surgical management, and fertility outcomes for women with endometrioma. Acta Obstetricia et Gynecologica Scandinavica. 2017;**96**(6):633-643

[16] Chia-Lin H, Chii-Shinn S, Liang-Ming L, et al. Effectiveness of ultrasound-guided aspiration and sclerotherapy with 95% ethanol for treatment of recurrent ovarian endometriomas. Fertility and Sterility. 2009;**91**:2709-2713

[17] Philip C-A, Warembourg S, Dairien M, et al. Transrectal high-intensity focused ultrasound (HIFU) for the management of rectosigmoid deep infiltrating endometriosis: Results of phase I clinical trial. Ultrasound in Obstetrics & Gynecology. 2019;**56**(3)